The Seen But Forgotten

An Insight into Mental Illness and the Dangers of Current Psychiatric Practice

I0117953

Victoria Musgrave

chipmunkapublishing
the mental health publisher

Victoria Musgrave

Published by
Chipmunkapublishing

http://www.chipmunkapublishing.com

Edited by Dru Impleton

The Seen But Forgotten

Gratefully dedicated to my friend, mentor and carer,
Peter Berther, whom without his support and ideas
related to some of its subject matter, would not have
been written.

Victoria Musgrave

The Seen But Forgotten

TABLE OF CONTENTS

About the Author   7

Book Description   11

Important Recommendation   13

Introduction   15

PART I   : What is mental health?   31

PART II   : The big picture: some possible causes of
mental illness   41

PART III : Paranoia   61

PART IV : Delusions   67

PART V   : Depression   71

PART VI : Schizophrenia: an inner hell and state of mind   77

PART VII : Medication therapy (the dangers)   85

PART VIII: The hope for recovery   95

PART IX : Conclusion   111

APPENDIX : Spirituality: the missing link in psychiatry?   127

Wisdom from the Dalai Lama - Meditations on the Family   130

References   131

Victoria Musgrave

About the Author

Victoria Musgrave is a Graduate Architect in Australia, and was born in 1966. She has suffered with mental illness now for nearly thirty years and would like to try to help and contribute to others, by sharing what she has learned as she continues to recover. As Victoria continually grows as a person, she would like to try to show others whom may be struggling with a mental health condition, how she managed to get quite a bit better, in the hope of perhaps reducing the suffering of another. Victoria graduated from the Queensland University of Technology in 1993, after seven years of study, with two Bachelor Degrees in Architecture and the Built Environment. This was despite being diagnosed with a serious mental illness in 1992.

Victoria was first diagnosed with schizophrenia in 1991, at twenty five years of age, after suffering a nervous breakdown when experiencing some severe life stressors, including a broken engagement to her then fiance of two and a half years. And she admits that she was "off her head". Victoria told her psychiatrist at the time that she was chosen to save the world. By 1993, as her life was spiralling out of control and she suffered from her first manic episode, her initial diagnosis was then changed to schizoaffective disorder, then incorporating the comorbid mood component of this illness, known as Bipolar Affective Disorder. Victoria has been in and out of hospitals ever since, both in the public and private mental health systems. It has taken her many years since then to learn about and work on her own personal journey of recovery, in order to be much more successful today, at fifty three years of age.

In writing "The Seen But Forgotten", Victoria found the process to be extremely therapeutic and cathartic, and would encourage interested persons to read her book, because she would like to help others whom have mental illness, and their families and carers, as well as try to inform researchers working on the medical treatments of mental illness, and nurses and psychiatrists where they are failing in some areas. The arguments and opinions put forward in her book are confronting and controversial, and upsetting to the status quo of current psychiatric practice. However, this has been done decidedly in an attempt to encourage more widespread awareness about the dangers of current psychiatric practice, and also encourage more debate. At times, the way that Victoria was treated and overmedicated for too long, nearly on so many occasions killed her. And she witnessed this happen to a lot of other patients with mental illness along the way too. Victoria even lost several friends to suicide during this time.

Victoria is very much more well today now that she has taken some control back of her life, and has been in recovery now for around seven years. This has mainly been achieved with help from psychiatrists and mental health nurses, and other mental health professionals, like psychologists, and also due to her own efforts and hard work. Victoria has also been on a personal spiritual journey, which for her has also provided a great deal of comfort, strength, hope and personal advancement. Over the past ten years or so Victoria has also been involved in collaborations, mostly on a volunteer basis, with a few non-government organisations designing conceptual proposals of supported accommodation for young people with schizophrenia, with the aim of these organisations obtaining funding to build much more of this type of much needed housing, to help house young adults with mental illness whom may be vulnerable to homelessness as their ageing parents become unable to continue to care for them.

Victoria Musgrave

Book Description

"The Seen But Forgotten: An Insight into Mental Illness and the Dangers of Current Psychiatric Practice", has been written based on nearly thirty years of experience of mental illness, "schizoaffective disorder" and anxiety, as well as on many of my observations and other ideas, and related research on mental illness. It is in part also based on observations of many of my friends and associates with mental illness over many years, and some of their stories and experiences relayed to me. It describes some insights into some of the thoughts and feelings one can experience in certain states of mental illness. It also offers an overview of both already known and other hypothetical considerations of some of the other possible causes of mental illness. It also includes some consideration of the medical model of the more current psychiatric practice of 'chemical drug therapy'. The dangers and sometimes errors of this practice is emphasized, and exposed are some of the serious and premature death-inducing side effects of a lot of psychiatric medications, the dangers associated with the overuse and misuse of benzodiazepines, and why there is a need for more research in new directions, in order for psychiatrists, medical researchers and pharmaceutical companies to come up with safer treatments.

Also discussed within my book are some suggestions for people with mental illness, carers and mental health workers about ways for one who is suffering from mental distress or illness to also try to help oneself and relieve some of their suffering, apart from relying solely on medication. It also includes a section about recovery, entitled "The Hope for Recovery", as well as the topic of recovery being discussed throughout other

11

sections of my book, including suggestions made in section entitled "Conclusion". Particular references are made here to some ideas related to recovery and schizophrenia, and which have helped me tremendously in my journey towards being more well, and more highly functioning again, as I was prior to the onset of my own mental illness.

The topic of 'spirituality' as the missing link in psychiatry is introduced briefly in a summary way in the Appendix at the end of my book, and makes reference to some of the work of other writers, including Jeremy Griffith and the Dalai Lama. The topic introduced in this section is considered as a whole other area in itself of too broad a scope to be discussed in too much detail, given our differing ideas and spiritual beliefs or leanings, and is not the main argument or purpose of my book here. Thus, it has been introduced in this way, as well as by suggestions in the sections 'The Hope for Recovery' and 'Conclusion', in the hope of encouraging further thought and consideration by the reader.

There is also at the end of my book, a list of references from where the technical, scientific, medical and psychoanalytic theories, information and terminology, has been derived to support the research to help support the argument and overall messages contained in my book.

IMPORTANT RECOMMENDATION:

Any person, having read this book, who decides to make any changes to or stop taking their medication prescribed for the treatment of a mental illness, should only do so under medical supervision and in consultation with their doctor. It is not recommended that you stop or make changes to your current medication regime without first embarking on your own recovery journey, including utilizing self-help strategies and assistance from your treating mental health professional.

The Author does not bear any responsibility for a person who does not seek professional advice.

The purpose of this book is not to encourage people with mental illness to stop their medication. Rather, it aims to promote more debate and discussion by those with mental illness and mental health professionals; and to suggest that research be done into safer and more holistic treatments for mental disorders.

I wish you well.

Victoria Musgrave

INTRODUCTION

According to recorded history, mental illness has existed in human beings since some of the earliest known times and since the advent of industrialization. Since this time, people with mental illness have been much maligned and misunderstood, and mistreated, institutionalized and hidden away from the rest of society. It has only been a relatively recent phenomenon where those with mental illness are being better understood, taken better care of and offered more help, and are treated with more dignity and respect. This has been indicated by the more recent advent of deinstitutionalization, since the 1980's, and as a result of the studies, research and hard work undertaken by psychiatrists, nurses, psychologists, case managers, and pharmaceutical scientists; and other allied medical field researchers. It has also been due to the fact that there are more people who have had a lived experience of mental illness and have recovered and are sharing insights, or are even still suffering from a mental illness, and are speaking out and being listened to better.

The study of mental illness is also now an area of psychiatry and psychology which is continually and progressively 'advancing', however, still not yet developing treatments which 'go back to basics' and treat the <u>root cause</u> and not just the symptoms, in order to promote prevention rather than treatments which often produce adverse side effects, obesity, over-sedation, and resultant early deaths from medical complications, and suicide. It seems that research is in its infancy and is still not headed in the best direction.

There is, in some instances, also a degree of corruption and cover-up going on today amongst the psychiatric associations and international drug companies. They have become industries created to support each other and make huge profits at the expense of the lives of some of the most vulnerable in our society. Psychiatrists, knowingly or not, mental hospitals and most of the drug treatments have, and still are in fact, killing innocent and already suffering people. Modern medicine cannot keep up with evolution and the microbiological world. For example, the constant updating of antibiotics for treatment resistant strains of bacteria (or 'super bugs') in diseases such as pneumonia and tuberculosis, are looked at as occurring in people with a 'genetic predisposition'. Similarly, this is how the occurrence of mental illness is also seen; as one having such a genetic predisposition. Doctors are starting to discover, though, that illnesses such as heart disease in fact have an infectious element (and not a genetic predisposition), that is, a bacteria in the blood, and exacerbated by factors like high blood cholesterol and smoking. There are also causes of mental illness, discussed further in *PART II*, however, environmental factors are more of a concern than researchers are really letting on thus far.

Concerning governments and the lack of adequate funding in Australia in mental health and mental health recovery programs (including supportive accommodation, rehabilitation, and employment for consumers), due to their self-serving hierarchy, the underlying truth is that they are not promoting a *duty of care* and sufficient funding to better help people with mental illness, who are at the lowest rung of the social ladder. This spotlights a major problem. However, there are many groups of people and organizations who are willing to, and actually are, working to help rectify this situation. "The paternalistic culture which exists is one where the repression of basic needs and functions becomes inevitable, (Stevens,1994). This could include the attitude and stigma still existing of governments towards people in society with mental illness. According to Stevens, this type of societal foundation is related directly to capitalism and alienated self interest, (greed, even corruption). Repression of basic needs, in Stevens' opinion, (such as 'love') does not stop where it begins. If we do not satisfy them naturally and well, then we take up substitutes often obsessively.

As part of the 'schizophrenic' reaction to the repression of such needs, behaviour will continue to create and promote 'madness', (especially it could be said, cause violence, wars and power mongers), (adapted from Stevens, 1994)."

There is no doubt that mental illness exists, this is not the issue. It is the treatments and ideas about it that are still somewhat primitive (baseless, perhaps even cruel). Some organizations, for example, drug companies, psychiatric fraternities, and government, become bigger and more important than those for whom they were originally set up to serve; usually because large amounts of money are involved. This leads to an element of gates to corruption. Some psychologists, psychiatrists and carers believe that mental illness can develop in people from loving families. This is certainly true, and there can still exist love in dysfunctional families. It is a difficult task to maintain a truly healthily-functioning family environment all of the time. However, sometimes one may think that theirs is a loving family because they do not know anything different; for example, as a result of conditioning, a sense of loyalty, personality type, denial, et cetera. Often, the development of mental illness, or mental health problems, depends on the amount of undue stress, trauma, or even abuse, that one has gone through in their life, and over what length of time this may have occurred for problems to develop.

According to Hillman, the Swiss psychiatrist Carl Jung (1875-1961) remarked:

The God's have become diseases. To see the angel in the malady requires an eye for the invisible, a certain blinding of one eye and an opening of the other to elsewhere. It is impossible to see the angel unless you first have a notion of it; otherwise the child is simply stupid, willful or pathological.

In the final analysis, we count for something only because of the essential we embody, and if we do not embody that, life is wasted (Hillman, 1996).

Having a mental illness can be one of the most debilitating and frightening experiences that a person can face. The intense suffering involved in the experiences of the different types of mental illness for the sufferers should not ever be trivialized. There is still the associated stigma from society in general, a lack of understanding by most people, a loss of being able to function for the person with a mental illness and a substantially lessened quality of life for the person whilst they are still unwell. Worse still, sometimes when one can see no way out of their pain or does not have access to good help, suicide can be attempted and is often successful. In many cases, psychiatric drugs simply compound the problem. Some of the side effects can be severe, for example, especially from ingesting anti-psychotic drugs, that the person forced to take them gets worse and attempts suicide, often succeeding.

The Seen But Forgotten

Understanding the *thoughts and feelings* and the terrible fears of someone in the midst of anxiety disorders, psychosis, depression, hallucinations or paranoia for example, is of paramount importance for carers and mental health professionals. This is needed to be able to empathize with the person and help him or her to feel safe. It is also important for mental health professionals to provide education to the person about their illness to try to help them to be able to gain some insight into their condition, utilizing only minimal doses of pharmaceutical drugs on a short term basis, whilst at the same time employing trained psychologists to provide counseling and therapy.

The general public and society also need to be made more aware and be better informed about the reality of the real human suffering of people with mental illness, in order to try to reduce stigma and better understand the trials and burdens that some of us have been handed. Mental illness is *not* a sign of weakness, nor is it a state of malingering. It can be as physical and as painful in essence as cancer or diabetes for example, and needs to be recognized and treated as such in order for society to be encouraged to help more and not hold too many unrealistic notions and fears about those of us who have mental illness. Many people are frightened of those who suffer with mental illness due to a fear that it could happen to them, and also because most people do not want to accept that others actually have mental illness. Therefore, the 'out of sight, out of mind' idea becomes very attractive to most of us. This ignorance, judgmental attitude and total lack of compassion and understanding then makes it even harder for people with mental illness to recover well and have a more normal life.

It seems that for some people, their mental illness becomes physical over time, worsening for the sufferer depending on their perceived level of alienation from society, other people, and their choices about what to do with their life. In order for insight to be gained, so that the person can attempt to be more mindful and improve their mental state, one needs to accept, for now, the realities of exclusion, alienation, misunderstanding from peers, and/or extraordinary abilities, which they may have experienced and accept themselves and their non-conventionality in the more common or more socially accepted way of life.

This book offers some brief explanations about what mental health is; what recovery from mental illness is; and insights in to some of the thoughts, the psychological world, and how it can feel in some states of mental illness. It also offers an overview of both some known and other hypothetical considerations of the possible causes of mental illness; some possible triggers from a psychoanalytic point of view; and also includes some critical consideration of the medical model of the current psychiatric practice of 'chemical drug therapy'. The dangers and error of this scenario is suggested, and exposed is the serious and premature death-inducing side-effects of most 'anti-psychotic' drugs created by the international drug companies, and why they need to be avoided and replaced with better treatments in order to be safe and to preserve life….not lead to unnecessary deaths.

Berther wrote about the treatment of persons "assumed to be suffering from a mental illness". The following excerpt is taken directly from his work:

Now that Kornelia Rau (after being misdiagnosed by the Princess Alexandra Hospital) has reportedly been compensated by a Federal government department for illegal incarceration, it follows that all persons suffering (or appearing to suffer from a mental illness), receive an apology from the Federal Government.

The Federal Government has ignored the pressing need for uniformity in the treatment of mental illness since Federation, and passed responsibility to the States, similar to Indigenous persons' treatment. Therefore. APOLOGY, COMPENSATION, and REHABILITATION FOR SURVIVORS must be addressed jointly by Federal and State departments.

May I suggest that compensation and rehabilitation for survivors in Queensland (Australia) *be effected by using the money that Queensland Housing has scammed from its tenants under lease agreements; to build, staff and maintain a Rehabilitation Township at "The Park"* (Wacol, Brisbane)*; Centre for Mental Health Research, Treatment and Education* (QCMHR)*. Other individual States and Territories will have to formulate their own systems for rehabilitation, because the Federal Government still refuses to admit that a NATIONAL MENTAL HEALTH ACT is imperative.*

The current alcohol problem with Indigenous communities throughout Australia originated in the Rumcorps of early settlements in New South Wales, and has been exacerbated by the granting of drinking rights to Indigenous communities. Australia's reputation for hard drinking habits is reflected in the teenage binge drinking mentality. Drugs, binge drinking, alcoholism and 'dual diagnosis' should not be grouped with mental illness. Those problems are caused by a combination of alcohol and social drugs which should be separated from the actual treatment of those who do suffer from a mental illness; the causes of which are mental and sexual abuse, acquired brain injury, and the genetics of incestual breeding, and our chemical society. Mental health consumers should not be subject to the behaviour problems of drug addicts and alcoholics who choose to fry their brains (Berther, 2007).

Further quotes from Berther's work about this subject are included in *PART IX: CONCLUSION.*

There are many causes for concern and necessary considerations to be made in one taking or changing antipsychotic medication. At present, as antipsychotic medications are being prescribed to treat psychotic features of mental illnesses like schizophrenia, schizoaffective disorder and bipolar affective disorder, any medication change-over needs to be very gradual, in order to minimize suffering and keep the person as comfortable as possible. The 'withdrawals', or discontinuation side effects, from reducing and eventually ceasing a previous medication can be difficult or distressing if done too rapidly. For example, some people experience restlessness or a 'stomping' of their feet and legs, increased anxiety and increased sweating. In addition, realizing the potential for a relapse or worsening of psychotic symptoms; during the period of time in which the newly introduced medication has not yet become therapeutic; is important to take into account and the patient be closely monitored in a hospital environment, and supported throughout this process by nursing staff.

It is prudent, when any change-over of antipsychotic medication is trialed, for this to be carried out in the hospital setting so that the patient can be helped to feel safe and protected. Monitoring is also important so that one's doctor and the nursing staff can watch out for and treat as soon as possible any adverse reactions or unwanted extrapyramidal side-effects of the new medication (or medications) being tried. This approach would help the patient to feel safer if a severe reaction did occur, and help to minimize their stress and anxiety levels. Help would be immediately available in this scenario.

Some of the potential side-effects of antipsychotic medications can be very painful and frightening, as well as fatal. These adverse reactions can even be more distressing than the illness for which they were originally prescribed to treat. Some examples of such extrapyramidal side-effects are:

➢ Akathisia, which is quite common; a state of mild to severe physical discomfort and restlessness where the person experiencing it can have great difficulty in sitting still, may exhibit rocking movements when able to sit, or has to pace up and down the floor because they cannot sit still. This reaction can be extremely distressing, and has precipitated many suicide attempts as well as led to actual suicides;

➢ Tardive dyskinesia, which can occur after long-term therapy with an antipsychotic medication, usually the older 'typical' antipsychotics. It is characterized by uncontrollable twitching or swinging of the legs, rapid blinking, lip-smacking, worm-like movements of the tongue, movement of the jaw from side to side and/or unusual facial grimacing. Tardive dyskinesia can be reversible, however, it can take months, or even years, for it to resolve itself once the receptors, neurons and chemicals in the brain return to normal functioning once the medication which caused it is ceased;

➢ Some other side effects of both the 'typical' and newer 'atypical' antipsychotic drugs include: slowing of voluntary movement, expressionless face, rigidity, tremor of the arms and head, abnormal toxicity of the muscle tissues, and restlessness;

➢ The most serious, but rare, adverse reaction (emphasizing why hospitalization should be recommended when changing-over or starting on an antipsychotic medication) is Neuroleptic Malignant Syndrome (NMS), a potentially fatal symptom complex which has been reported in association with the administration of antipsychotic drugs. Manifestations of NMS are 'hyperpyrexia', muscle rigidity, altered mental status, and evidence of autonomic instability (that is, irregular pulse or blood pressure, tachycardia, diasphoresis, and cardiac dysthmia), and acute renal failure;

➢ Some of the more recent 'atypical' antipsychotic drugs, such as 'clozaril' and 'zyprexa', can adversely affect blood glucose levels, trigger increased appetite which can lead to significant weight gain. This has, in some people, caused hyperglycemia (elevated blood sugar), diabetes mellitus, or an exacerbation of pre-existing diabetes, and cardiovascular disease associated with obesity (NARSAD, www.narsad.org, 2007).

Given this list of possible adverse reactions and side-effects of antipsychotic drugs, it may be obvious that long-term use can be dangerous. There continued use could be, in many cases, a path towards additional pain and unnecessary suffering. This is why it is so important for new research to be funded and undertaken into better ways of trying to treat the symptoms (and discover the causes) of mental illness, whilst at the same time inviting more psychotherapy and counseling into the equation to promote growth and recovery. The human animal is a complex being, and it takes more than just drugs to supposedly correct a chemical imbalance in the brain when trying to help people heal and get better from a mental health issue or problem.

Apart from the negative effects of taking antipsychotic medications ('major' tranquilizers), the benzodiazepine anti-anxiety class of drugs (or 'minor' tranquilizers), such as 'valium' (diazepam) and 'serepax' (oxazepam), are also fraught with serious problems with prolonged use. These are not involving fatality problems, as for the antipsychotic class of medications; however, they can lead to a whole lot of unnecessary suffering and addiction when not used properly. This class of medications are very useful for a person in a crisis, and do work very well with short-term use. Prolonged use, or the administrating of very high doses, however, is often harmful and does not actually remove the root cause of one's stress or anxiety. The incorrect prescribing and use of minor tranquilizers can create more problems and anxiety (rebound anxiety) in the long run with prolonged overuse and lack of monitoring of use by the prescribing physician.

The more recent situation whereby some prescribing doctors, as well as nurses in the hospital environment (and, often even patients), still do not understand the dangerous addictive properties of the benzodiazepine class of drugs, and continue to over-prescribe and administer them, is both regrettable and a cause for concern. Often the person taking these medications, believing that they are safe and are helping relieve their anxiety, can find himself, after some time (perhaps only a few weeks) taking even higher doses to attempt to get the same level of relief from their anxiety as before. However, they instead find that their anxiety is escalating without really understanding why. It often takes, after some time, an even higher dose of such drugs to achieve the same effect as that received previously after one has been taking the drug for too long. Thus, a drug dependency situation has been created and the person can become quite desperate and unwell, and experience a lot worse anxiety than they had had before they first started taking a benzodiazepine medication (Wilkie, 1985). Where the problem may be recognized early enough by a person's doctor, it is often the case whereby a carefully planned and medically supervised withdrawal regime is required to help the person who is 'hooked' to gradually taper off the drug. This, depending on the length of time someone has been taking a benzodiazepine, can be a long, hard and traumatic experience. The person can, in withdrawal, suffer many extremely frightening, painful and distressing symptoms. This withdrawal is a series of physical, psychological and behavioural changes experienced when a drug is cut down or ceased. From research, it has been established that it is likely that fifty to eighty per cent of people who have taken benzodiazepines for six months or longer will experience withdrawal (*About Withdrawal-What is Happening to Me?*, Alcohol and Drug Information Service, 2003).

Benzodiazepine withdrawal symptoms usually appear in clusters and affect the hormonal, immune and metabolic systems. Common symptoms include excessive sweating, nausea, dizziness, blurred vision, anxiety, panic attacks, depression, suicidal thoughts, and insomnia. For many people, the intensity of withdrawal symptoms is overwhelming, although it varies from person to person. Withdrawal can take many weeks, months or (for some people) even years. Usually the length of time a person has been taking benzodiazepines, or the amount he or she has been taking, will have the most impact on the time it takes to come off the drug. Generally, the longer the body has been accustomed to functioning with the drug, the longer the withdrawal will take (*About Withdrawal and its Symptoms-What is Happening to Me?* Alcohol and Drug Information Service, 2003).

An uncomplicated withdrawal from a benzodiazepine will usually only last for a few weeks. However, the withdrawal symptoms may continue for many months, or even up to one year. For some people, withdrawal symptoms last even longer than two to three years, where they have been taking the drug for a very long time. It can take a long time during this syndrome for the body to return to its previous normal chemically balanced state.

When used for too long a period of time, benzodiazepine drugs can act as a depressant, and can dampen and suppress one's emotions and ability to think clearly and rationally. This lack of mental alertness can also rob a person of motivation and their ability or resolve to be able to cope or help themselves. And, their abrupt withdrawal (ceasing 'cold turkey') can be dangerous and very distressing due to the possibility of having seizures, or other symptoms like extreme restlessness in the legs. Abuse of these medications is all too insidiously and mistakenly easy, often with devastating consequences, especially when the person who has become dependent does not understand why they feel so stressed, tense and anxious.

With the use of benzodiazepines, as well as other psychotropic medications like antipsychotic drugs and antidepressants, for some people who are being treated for a mental illness, they can sometimes develop a great degree of apathy. That is, not only do the drugs become a 'habit', life itself and poor mental health also becomes a habit. This is, in many cases, because more holistic approaches to treating mental illness have not been adopted by the medical profession in a lot of areas. It seems that to some 'patients' that the way of life of 'popping pills' is as good as it going to get. The drugs become a habit and way of life, and such lack of motivation and ability to recover becomes a tragic outcome for many people with mental illness, where their lives end up not really being lived.

Overuse of medications can also increase the 'negative' symptoms of one's mental condition, such as lack of motivation and the apathy often noticed in people who suffer with schizophrenia and clinical depression. This is because the person on medication has become drugged on too heavy doses of medication, which contributes to the 'laziness' and lack of a sense of purpose in participating in life and being alive. Here, sadly, mental wellness can allude this class of consumers for years, even for the rest of their life, until they can (or are given the opportunity to) better help themselves and do the work which is necessary in order to recover. The medical model of treatment has made this venture more difficult by introducing an overemphasis on drug treatments and not enough attention paid to the psychological counseling approach. As it is now widely established that genes and childhood environment go hand in hand in contributing to mental illnesses, like depression, bipolar disorder and schizophrenia, more psychological 'talk' therapy can be undertaken as early as possible to help the sufferer to get back to wellness, or at least manage their condition as best as they can. This can only serve to increase a person's quality of life and help create for them increased opportunities for 'normality': such as to be able to work, have meaningful relationships, and pursue their goals and aspirations.

It would be useful to consider: what makes up a person; on their intellectual, emotional, physical and spiritual levels? These categories would need to be taken into account in any 'treatment' for their mind (and body and soul). One would need to consider and describe also: what is good mental health for a person, and if one develops mental illness, how can they get back to good mental health, or at least recover as much as possible?

Mental health is, of course, an important component of overall health and wellbeing. However, sometimes external and environmental factors, such as unexpected events and traumas, occur that affect our mental (and physical) health. The following section: *PART I: What is Mental Health?*, looks at what makes up poor mental health and good mental health, and describes some ways in which one can maintain good mental health, even despite the presence of mental illness.

Victoria Musgrave

PART I

WHAT IS MENTAL HEALTH?

One could say that we are our thoughts, plans, ideas and emotions. However, these cannot exist in a 'mental vacuum'. Can we control our own destiny based on intuition or gut instincts? (Goleman, 1996). Ours, perhaps, *is* to reason why, and there may be a deeper purpose for existence that not one of us really yet fully understands. For those who struggle and attempt to make the world a better place, it can hurt to grow. Perhaps, though, facing pain is not nearly as terrible as avoiding it; when you can come out the other side better and stronger for having been through a challenge or difficult time and coped successfully.

For those who do not care, are greedy, competitive and have only eyes for a material-oriented world, how much can they truly learn about life and see what is going on around them; yet passively reject opportunities to do anything about it? In the so-called 'advanced' Western world, we are living in an increasingly spiritless society, developing at an ever-increasing pace, with the advancement of technology leaving behind moral values. This rapid rate of change is also placing too much pressure on today's parents and children. Often, poor mental health, even mental illness, can result from the whole range of consequences of society developing too quickly and forgetting to nurture one's body, mind and soul in the process.

Good mental health is not just the absence of mental illness. Good mental health is also not an absolute concept, as some people are more mentally healthy than others, whether they suffer from a mental illness or not. Mental health is a core component of psychological wellbeing, and, therefore, everyday life is as important as physical health. This distinguishes the concept of 'mental health' from the numerous types of clinically diagnosable 'mental illnesses'; such as anxiety, depression, bipolar disorder, schizophrenia, schizoaffective disorder, personality disorders, and eating disorders.

According to the Canadian Mental Health Association website (www.cmha.ca), in considering the meaning of mental health, the following characteristics were regarded as important in gauging your own mental health:

- **Ability to enjoy life**- *i.e. can you live in the moment and appreciate the 'now'? Are you able to learn from the past and plan for the future without dwelling on things you cannot change or predict?*
- **Resilience**- *i.e. are you able to bounce back from hard times? Can you manage the stress of a serious life event without losing your optimism and a sense of perspective?*
- **Balance**- *i.e. are you able to juggle the many aspects of your life? Can you recognize when you may be devoting too much time to one aspect, at the expense of others? Are you able to make changes to restore balance when necessary?*
- **Self-actualization**- *i.e. do you recognize and develop your strengths so that you can reach your full potential?*
- **Flexibility**- *i.e. do you feel, and express, a range of emotions? When problems arise, can you change your expectations - of life, others, and yourself – to solve the problem and feel better?*

All human beings have varying opinions, attitudes, physical health and mental health. As with physical health, a person's mental health can range from good to poor. It is now widely established by researchers that good mental health is essential to overall good physical health; and that our physical and mental health are connected. As it is in today's society that some are misjudged because of race, ethnicity, religion or culture; people with mental illness can also be treated unfairly, especially in regards to things such as appropriate housing, employment, education, treatment, and biased media attention.

Stigma and discrimination from others is still a real issue in society and can be very harmful to the lives of people with mental illness. The shame associated with stigma may prevent some people from getting treatment and the support that they need to lead to healthier, more normal lives. Stigma also has often led to fear and mistrust of the mentally ill person, which serves to alienate them from family and others. The resulting bias, where some people try to prevent those with a mental illness from living in their neighbourhood, for example, also shows a lack of understanding and acceptance.

As poor physical health may increase the likelihood of developing poor mental health, poor mental health may increase the risks of developing, or not recovering from, serious physical health problems. Whilst good mental health is an important part in successful psychological and social functioning, poor mental health has been associated with poor socio-economic status, poor education and lack of opportunities for employment, and a range of inequalities, some of which fall under the umbrella term 'social exclusion'. Mental health issues can range from common problems such as 'feeling depressed' to more severe problems, such as 'clinical depression' and more lasting problems such as 'schizophrenia'. These are just two examples of diagnosable and/or clinical levels of mental health problems.

Mental health problems have usually been categorized in two major ways:

- *Organic (an identifiable brain malfunction) versus functional (not due to structural abnormalities of the brain); and*
- *Neurosis (severe forms of normal experiences such as low mood and anxiety) versus psychosis (severe distortions of a person's perception of reality)*

(The Mental Health Foundation, Mental Health Problems, fact sheet, London, 2003).

The latter definition is usually classed as being a form of mental illness, set apart from the meaning of 'mental health' as described above.

Therefore, regardless of the type of mental health problem a person may experience; organic conditions, functional, neurotic and psychotic mental conditions require different types of medical and psychological treatments, and effort on the part of the person themselves in order for them to have the best mental health outcome as possible. This involves being able to participate in work, relationships and life to the best of one's ability despite having problems or mental health issues or mental illness.

The diagram shown of a *Model of a Person* illustrates those main parts of a person which go to make up their whole self: on the intellectual (or mind) level; and the physical, emotional and spiritual levels. These four major components need to have certain needs and preferences met in order for a person to experience good mental health, where basic life requirements are satisfied and enjoyment is gained; or poor mental health (and/or physical health) where needs are not met, or unhealthy actions and behaviours are indulged in. An example for the latter scenario is engaging in risky behaviour such as taking illicit drugs or drinking too much alcohol. It is widely known today that these types of activities can lead to poor physical health and mental health problems.

In using our intellect (or mind), we are able to engage in activities, such as work, in order to aim to be fulfilled and get a sense of achievement and contentment. It is often that when opportunities for recreational activities arise, like going to the movies, we enjoy this time for fun more-so after working, as it becomes well-earned and is felt as a reward. This type of engagement of the intellect is often a healthy one, as it can also assist in us getting needs met on the physical and emotional levels as well.

MODEL OF A PERSON

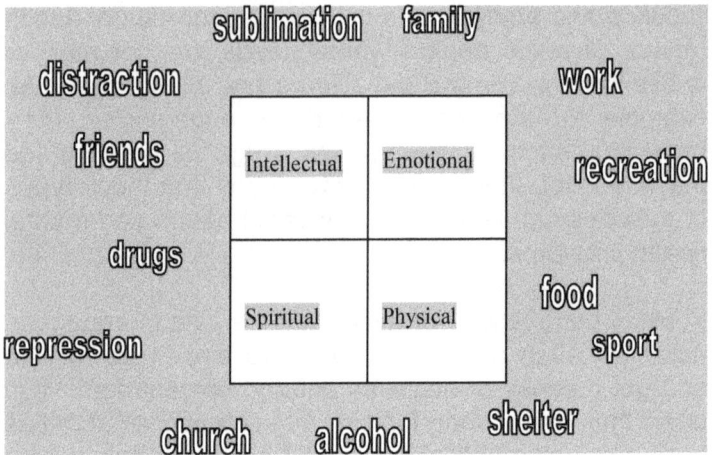

The body needs to be physically healthy, that is, be free from illness or disease, and have its basic needs of: enough food and water; adequate shelter; clothing and warmth; and medical intervention or assistance as a prevention measure; satisfied, to help promote overall wellbeing. In regards to the emotional aspects of ourselves, good mental and physical health is gained by having enough love, affection, and meaningful and rewarding relationships, especially from one's family, relatives, friends and a significant other for most people. Spiritual (or religious) beliefs are also very significant and important to many people's lives and sense of wellbeing; in providing direction, purpose, love, clarity for some, and meaning. The feeling that one's journey may have meaning, especially during hard times or emotional upheaval, can help a person to be stronger and cope with the many adversities in life that can occur. For some people, a spiritual or religious path does help them and can provide comfort, direction and be good for one's mental and emotional health.

The Seen But Forgotten

A mental health issue or problem comes from a lack of *balance* in the satisfaction of the basic needs of the four components of what makes a person, as shown in the diagram above. A mental illness is a health problem that significantly affects how a person thinks, behaves and interacts with other people. It is diagnosed according to certain standardized criteria. Good mental health is a sense of well-being, confidence and self-esteem. It enables people to fully enjoy and appreciate other people, day-to-day life and our environment. When we have good mental health we can: *form positive relationships, use our abilities to reach our potential, and deal with life's challenges* (www.health.wa.gov.au/mentalhealth, 2008).

According to the Western Australian Government Department of Health:

Mental illness results from complex interactions between the mind, body and environment. Factors which can contribute to mental illness are:

- *Long-term and acute stress*
- *Biological factors, such as genetics, chemistry and hormones*
- *Use of alcohol, drugs and other substances*
- *Cognitive patterns, such as constant negative thinking and low self-esteem*
- *Social factors, such as isolation, financial problems, family breakdown or violence* (www.health.wa.gov.au/mentalhealth, 2008).

Therefore, in maintaining good mental health, one can attempt to minimize undue stress; only drink alcohol in moderation; avoid illicit drugs and other substances; try to limit negative-thinking; build positive self-esteem; try to find like-minded friends, family members and colleagues to interact with socially; minimize financial burdens by not living beyond one's means; and simply do the best that one can given the particular circumstances of one's life.

In Wilkie's understanding of will power, this is a function of the reticular activating system of the brain stem. This is made up of a network of cells and connecting fibers situated in the lower part of the brain, where the upper end of the spinal chord meets the brain's hemispheres. This is the activating system which makes us sleep at night and wake in the morning. It is also responsible for SELECTIVE ATTENTION, allowing us to concentrate on specific tasks, while excluding other sensory stimulus from our conscious awareness (Wilkie, 1985). Could this be linked in some way to what is termed by clinicians as *over-inclusive thinking* in people with schizophrenia or bipolar disorder, where some 'brilliant' minds have difficulty filtering out too much incoming sensory information in order to be able to better focus on what is more relevant at a particular time? Rapid speech, flights of ideas, thought disorder and the like are considered to be a form of sickness. Perhaps with the development of insight in people who tend to over-think, they could attempt to control it by the use of will power, education, therapy and training, rather than forcing 'zombie-like' states by opting too much for the use of medications, to give such a person a better quality of life. Wilkie also described how over-activation of parts of the cerebral cortex in the brain can induce a protective shut-down of such over-stimulated areas, resulting from *stress breakdown.*

The following section, *PART II*, discusses in an over-view fashion; some possible causes of mental illness, including those which are already established as agreed causes, as well as other hypothetical considerations about what also may cause mental illness.

PART II

THE BIG PICTURE: SOME POSSIBLE CAUSES OF MENTAL ILLNESS

If levels of neurotransmitter substances in the brain become diminished, it is shown from studies that it is possible that one's mood and behavior can become adversely affected.

Victoria Musgrave

The Nervous System and Behavior

NEURON A **NEUROTRANSMITTER SUBSTANCE** **NEURON B**

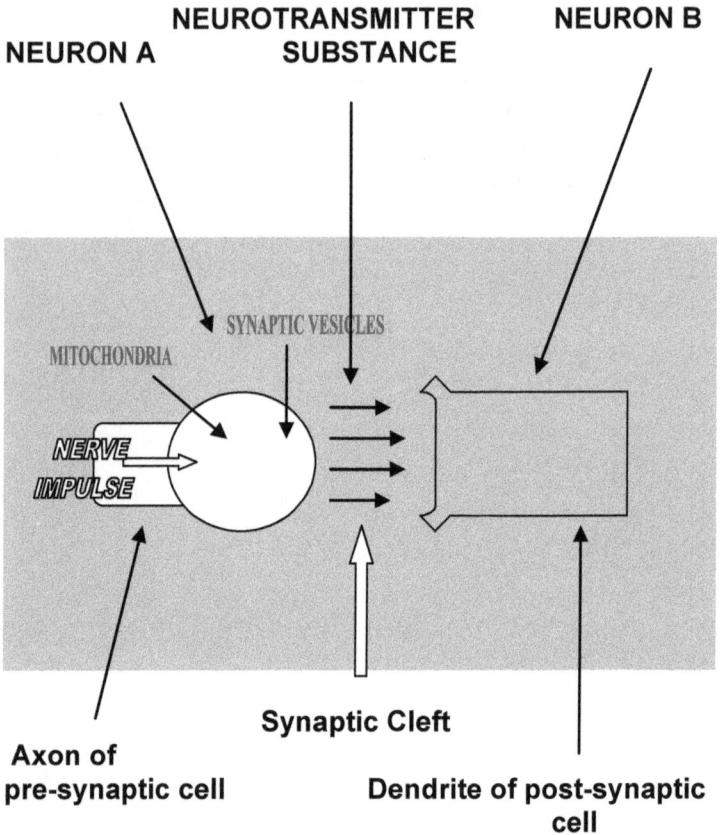

SYNAPTIC VESICLES

MITOCHONDRIA

NERVE IMPULSE

Synaptic Cleft

Axon of pre-synaptic cell

Dendrite of post-synaptic cell

(Electrical/chemical transmission process)
DIAGRAM OF A SYNAPSE

(Adapted from Taylor et al, 1982)

The Seen But Forgotten

The 'synaptic cleft' as illustrated in the diagram above showing a synapse and the nerve endings between the receptors in the human brain, is bridged by chemical transmitter molecules released by the synaptic vesicles inside the end of Neuron A.

The mitochondria provide the energy for the whole process of transmission via an electrical-chemical process, to carry messages from Neuron A to Neuron B through various neurotransmitter substances (Taylor et al, 1982).

Several different types of neurotransmitter substances have been found in the nervous system, some of which are:

(1) **EXCITATORY-** raising the probability of firing-off the post-synaptic cell (such as acetylcholine, glutamic acid, noradrenaline and norepinephrine); while others are:

(2) **INHIBITORY-** lowering the probability of firing-off the post-synaptic cell in their effects (such as acetylcholine, serotonin, dopamine, gamma aminobutyric acid and noradrenaline) (Taylor et al, 1982).

It has also been shown that changes in the levels of neurotransmitter substances available to be secreted at nerve endings can affect brain function. Therefore, it is highly likely that an INHIBITORY RESERVE reflects levels of available neurotransmitters (Wilkie, 1985).

The inhibitory reserve may be affected by the following factors, which may lead to either under-stimulation or over-stimulation of the brain's electrical/chemical function:

- Too much stress, such as, over-conditioning or suppression by guardians or parents when one is a child. The early environment and parent-child relationships in highly dysfunctional families can also lead to some maladaptive learned behaviors as the child grows into adulthood;
- Biological and genetic factors, especially if one is predisposed to a mental illness when it already exists in their family of origin;
- Emotional upsets and trauma, for example, sexual abuse and/or incest in families;
- Short electrical waves (electronic radiation) interfering with the brain's natural electrical and chemical energy and process, for example, due to excessive exposure to electrical waves from radio towers and mobile phones;
- Pollution and chemicals e.g. carbon emissions, toxins from food additives and preservatives, insecticides and other poisons, certain vaccinations, and some building materials etc. leading to neurotoxins, allergies and chemical reactions in the brain (and body);
- Alcoholism and illicit drug-taking, which affects very badly and kills brain cells;
- Obstetric complications at birth, for example resulting in nerve damage to the new born infant's brain as a result of instrument-assisted birth or other physical head trauma at birth; or other stress-induced neuro-chemical effects, such as a virus transmitted across the placenta from the mother to the fetus in utero;
- Toxic substances in the blood, such as beta endorphin (which is one proposed theory for a cause of schizophrenia);
- Personality type and painful psychological states such as inner conflicts, unmet needs and wishes,

thwarted drives, intentions and goals for one's life, repression of basic needs, or double bind situations; and

- Spiritual and psychological upset, also due to a lack of fulfillment, coupled with troubling societal or family pressures and expectations.

Could any of the above cause physical and electrical imbalances in the brain, and possibly lead to various mental disorders, such as, schizophrenia, schizoaffective disorder, bipolar disorder, major depression, and exacerbate, or even create, any of the personality disorders?

Within the medical model of attempting to find out more about the causes of mental illness, modern medicine is trying to find out why at a CELLULAR level, when levels of necessary neurotransmitter substances become diminished, affecting brain function in order to introduce chemical therapy. It has been suggested that the imbalance of these neurotransmitters can then affect:

- THOUGHTS
- EMOTIONS (OR FEELINGS)
- SENSES
- MOOD
- BEHAVIOUR
- DRIVE
- REACTIONS (OR EMOTIONAL RESPONSES) TO EVENTS
  (Bullock et al, 1997)

It can even be the case with this scenario that there appears to be a change in a person's PERSONALITY.

The question which has been hotly debated though is: Is mental illness really only genetic or physical in origin? Or, can the chemicals in the brain also become imbalanced after too much stress or other environmental trigger? It is understood that a genetic predisposition from one's biological parents almost certainly contributes towards a person developing a mental illness, and that genes and environment both play a part. Science is currently trying to isolate the specific genes which are thought to also play a big part in one developing a mental illness, in order to try to come up with better treatments and outcomes for sufferers.

According to ANALYTIC PSYCHOLOGY, man seeks *creative development, wholeness and completion* (Bullock et al, 1997). If this is suppressed in sensitive or gifted individuals, can they become so frustrated that they get mentally unwell as a result? As previously mentioned, upbringing and societal expectations in more vulnerable young developing individuals, can lead to a lack of fulfillment and despair in some cases.

The famous Swiss psychiatrist C. G. Jung (1875-1961) argued that an individual's functioning is the product of the COLLECTIVE UNCONCIOUS*, as well as of a PERSONAL UNCONSCIOUS, whose contents is forgotten, repressed, subliminally perceived *thought and felt* matter of every kind, and which, therefore, is not to be equated with the 'unconscious' of Freudian theory (Bullock et al, 1997).

Sigmund Freud (1856-1939) was a physiologist, medical doctor, psychologist and founder of psychoanalysis, and is generally recognized as one of the most influential and authoritative thinkers of the twentieth century. Working initially with Joseph Breuer, Freud put forward the theory that the mind is a complex energy-system, of which the structural investigation is fundamental to psychology. Freud described and refined the concepts of the 'unconscious', of infantile sexuality, of repression. He proposed a tri-partite theory of the mind's structure (the id, ego and super-ego), as part of a very new concept and therapeutic frame of reference for the supposed understanding of human psychological development and the treatment of mental illness. Despite the many manifestations of psychoanalysis that exists today, it can in many aspects be traced directly back to Freud's work. Freud's treatment of human actions, dreams, and also of cultural artifacts as having implicit symbolic significance has proven to be extremely prolific. It has had massive implications for a wide variety of fields of thought, including anthropology, semiotics, and artistic creativity and appreciation, as well as psychology. However, Freud's most important and often re-iterated claim to fame, that with psychoanalysis he had invented a new science of the mind, remains the subject of much critical debate and controversy (Thornton, 2006).

The psychologist Karen Horney (1883-1952) accepted REPRESSION and confused, blocked aims and wishes in personality development. She regarded unconscious factors as relevant only in more extreme neurosis and regarded social and interpersonal relationships as a more widespread source of stress and anxiety. Horney believed in the *primacy of anxiety* in the human experience (Bullock et al, 1997).

Brian imaging studies have shown that the parts of the brain, the AMYGDALA and NEOCORTEX, regulate feelings of anxiety (Goleman, 2003). In cases when a person is suffering from extreme anxiety, even to the point of becoming paranoid, or even driving psychosis, can this state also affect thoughts and emotions so adversely that one may also develop incongruous reactions to events and other people? It is the case in schizophrenia that a common symptom is where the sufferer has developed an incongruity between their thoughts and emotions, displaying odd behaviors to observers. A well documented and well known example of this is when the person suffering from schizophrenia may giggle or laugh at a gathering for a sad occasion such as a funeral, and where the reaction is considered inappropriate to others.   The state of mind of 'schizophrenia' is discussed in more depth in *PART VI* and attempts to explain how and why this state of mind can develop.

*The 'collective unconscious' is the Jungian term for past experience of the human species, which has been built in to the inherited brain structure and which manifests itself in the recurrent phenomena of ARCHETYPES, that is memories of one's ancestral history within the individual personality.

The 'unconscious' in psychoanalytic theory is the hypothesis that there are mental processes which operate outside of the individual's awareness, and which may play a key role in his or her life and in the explanation of BEHAVIOUR , whether it be 'a slip of the tongue' (commonly referred to as a Freudian slip) or a neurosis (Bullock et al, 1997).

Human functioning is much more goal-directed than we ordinarily suppose. Hence, this concept emphasizes the motivation of human THOUGHT and BEHAVIOUR, and prescribes that we look for the unconscious motives that on the unconscious, go to explain and determine our <u>conduct.</u>

The Seen But Forgotten

The EROS, our 'life instinct', in psychoanalytic theory, is a Freudian term for the supposed source of all the impulses and drives that serve the individual in self-preservation and reproduction. It is contrasted with the 'death instinct' (Thanatos) (Bullock et al, 1997).

If a child's or young adult's life instinct is repressed or suppressed by society, a parenting style, environment or others, can this affect or influence future thought, emotion and behavior in a detrimental way to the point of the child or young adult developing a mental illness? One's thoughts do help to create one's life or destiny. Emotions are felt as a subjective experience inferred from a complex set of behaviors, for example, from actions, facial expressions, movement and verbal communications. Behavioral disturbances, such as social withdrawal and loss of drive, can come from low self-esteem (and a perceived loss of potential in life) and depression and vice-versa, and even 'projection' where the person unconsciously blames others for their lack of self worth.

Anxiety, according to psychoanalytic theory (and necessary for survival) is both an emotional state and a trait of character. As with emotion, it is often used synonymously with FEAR- to fears whose object is not known. It can also be a state elicited by signals of impending punishment. As with a trait of character, it describes different degrees of susceptibility to fear. According to H.J. Eysenck, this trait is not unitary, but a composite of NEUROTICISM and INTROVERSION (Bullock et al, 1997).

Some standard emotional reactions incorporate elements of biologically-determined responses, while others are almost entirely socio-culturally determined. In 'transcendental emotional states', such as with anxiety, thinking becomes disorganized. With arousing stimuli, that is, either pleasant or unpleasant, anxiety increases and both levels of adrenaline (a hormone) and noradrenaline (a neurotransmitter) excretion increases (Taylor et al, 1982). The lack of connection between mental functions arising in the brain is an interesting field of study which has been considered and is being studied by doctors and scientists, with new information being discovered progressively.

It is now well established that schizophrenia causes disruption in the way different areas of the brain communicate with each other, and the disruption between the 'thinking' area of the prefrontal cortex and the 'feeling' area of the amygdala has come under special scrutiny. It is thought that neural disconnections between these two and other areas account for many of the disabilities associated with the illness. The reversal of connectivity between the feeling and thinking centers of the brain may be the root cause of the emotional alienation and social dysfunction symptomatic of schizophrenia (Newsletter, Schizophrenia Fellowship of Queensland Inc., 2007).

Freud was initially very pleased by attracting followers of the intellectual caliber of Adler and Jung around the time of his 1923 work on the tripartite model of the mind ('*The Ego and the Id*'). However, he was also personally disappointed when Adler and Jung both went on to found rival schools of psychoanalysis, which gave rise to the first two of many schisms in the movement. Freud considered that such disagreement over basic principles had been part of the early development of every new science (Thornton, 2006).

Freud's account of the unconscious, and the psychoanalytic therapy associated with it, is best illustrated by his tripartite model of the structure of the mind (or personality) shown in the 'iceberg' diagram; and which has many similarities with the account of the mind offered by Plato over two thousand years earlier. The *id*, Freud considered, is that part of the mind in which there are the instinctual sexual drives which require satisfaction; and the *super-ego,* that part which contains the 'conscience', usually imparted in the first instance by one's parents as socially-acquired control mechanisms, which have been internalized. The *ego*, Freud considered is the conscious self created by the dynamic tensions and interactions between the *id* and the *super-ego*, which has the task of reconciling their conflicting demands with the requirements of external reality (Thornton, 2006).

ICEBERG METAPHOR DIAGRAM OF FREUD'S CONCEPT OF THE MIND (PSYCHE)

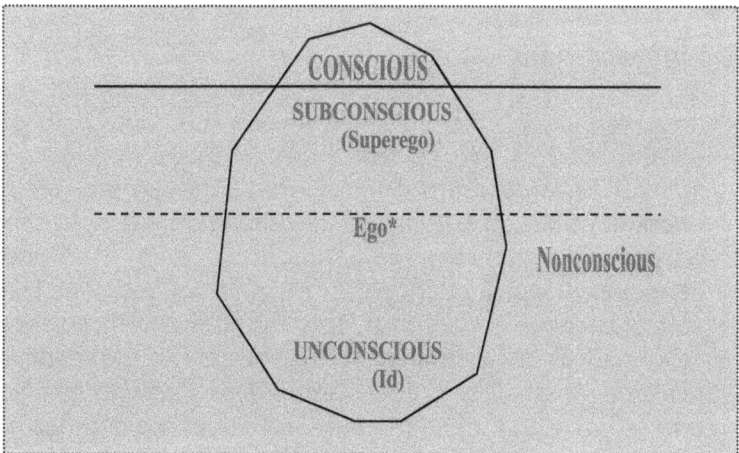

*The ego moves between all three levels

(Adapted from www.allpsych.com/psychology101/defenses.html, 2004) In relation to the subject of anxiety within models of personality and other psycho-dynamic theories, it has been suggested that the *ego* is often threatened by impulses from the *id*, as well as by external dangers in the environment, and when this happens anxiety occurs. Freud regarded anxiety as a regular and powerful source of pain which played a basic role in the organization of the person.

Anxiety became a topic of central importance during a later period for Freud. He became interested in the ways in which the ego is protected against acute anxiety resulting from conflict between rival impulses and postulated a number of defense strategies. In this later theory REPRESSION is one such strategy. It is a sort of 'amnesia' for avoiding the conscious experience of threatening impulses, wishes, memories, associations and motives (Bullock et al, 1997).

Another defense strategy is PROJECTION in which an anxiety-provoking impulse or emotion is attributed to another person. For example, if one has spite against another person, one comes to see that person as being spiteful towards them and others. The person feels uncomfortable, but it is less disturbing to attribute the unpleasant attributes to somebody else. Freud considered many such defenses and argued that the sort of defense a person adopts for coping with anxiety produced by conflict is an important clue to personality (Bullock et al, 1997). It often feels better to blame others for a lack of self-worth. However, sometimes a past trauma or even abuse of some kind has occurred for the person who is projecting for them to lack self-esteem, and to start to project.

Freud also made a distinction between the abovementioned two different types of behavior, and the super-ego:

(1) *The id is the product of HEREDITY and is the instinctual level of response. It is the main source of mental energy and is concerned with self-preservation, reproduction and aggression against threats. The primitive tensions and NEEDS of the id demand discharge in some kind of activity, if only <u>fantasies</u>.*

(2) *The ego is those activities of the brain which express themselves in intelligent actions. Whatever the primitive wishes of the id, reality must prevail. The ego-functions adjust or inhibit more primitive impulses to the complicated requirements of the SOCIAL ENVIRONMENT.*
(Bullock et al, 1997).

If the needs of the id are not met, can one become delusional due to delving too much into fantasy and unrealistic wishes and desires resulting from upset? Perhaps some people fail to learn to be able to inhibit impulses which fail to be adaptive or in touch with reality, especially when they refuse to or cannot adjust well to their social environment. This could be due to many factors, for example, from being placed in double bind situations or consistently being subject to emotional blackmail.

The ego and id often conflict. This can bring on mental stress and anxiety, and perhaps even sense deception?

The capacities of the ego-function to control a person are precarious and limited. The ego cannot always rule and compromise between conflicting tendencies can produce vacillating adaptations or maladaptive coping mechanisms, according to Freud (Bullock et al, 1997).

(3) The super-ego is a refinement of the ego function. It defines the values accepted by a person as a result of identifying with parents in childhood, and later modifying these on a basis of social experience (Bullock et al, 1997).

Therefore, it would be valid to reinforce the fact that our early environment influences our value system. However, we can later separate out some of those values and choose to no longer accept, believe or adopt them when they do not fit a later view or views about ourselves or our lives as we grow older.

At the root of our values, according to Freud, are very primitive emotions of FEAR and GUILT acquired in childhood during the 'Oedipus Crisis'*. Hence, the super-ego can be as irrational and impulsive as the id in prompting responses which threaten the ego, and so provoke anxiety. The ego-functions control and refine the promptings of the super-ego, and so produce sophisticated and rational moral values out of cruder material. Conflicts can be engendered in this process, which are as stressful as those from the functioning id-system. Thus in Freud's later thinking ego-functioning and its way of coping with anxiety was important and constituted a change in the theory.
*The 'Oedipus Crisis' is, in psychoanalytic theory, the normal emotional crisis brought about, at an early stage of psychosexual development, by the sexual impulses of a boy towards his mother and jealousy of his father. Resultant guilt feelings precipitate the development of the SUPEREGO (conscience). The female counterpart is the ELECTRA COMPLEX.

Repression is considered in psychoanalytic theory as a Freudian term which is used largely to refer to two distinct processes. These are namely:

(1) **PRIMAL REPRESSION:** *Where an infant or a child defends itself against the threat of excessive tension by attaching energy to some object or activity, where the energy functions antithetically, or counter, to the threatening tension.*

(2) **ACTUAL REPRESSION (OR REPRESSION PROPER):** *When an adult is threatened by the excessive tension that might arise if some unconscious wish, or impulse, moved into consciousness. This danger is signaled by anxiety, and it is met in various ways, for example, by withdrawing energy from the idea or thought of the threatening impulse so that it cannot move in to consciousness, rather it remains unconscious. Actual repression in Freudian theory is considered as a function of the Ego and unconscious in its operation* (Bullock et al, 1997).

A DEFENCE MECHANISM is also a Freudian term for any number of unconscious techniques or devices used by the ego to avoid danger, which is signaled by anxiety. There is no single agreed list of defense mechanisms, but the following techniques would usually be said to include:

(1) **IDENTIFICATION:** *In Social Psychology, the process of associating oneself closely with other individuals or reference groups to the extent that one comes to adopt their goals and*

values, and to share vicariously in their experiences. An example is peer groups;

(2) **PROJECTION** (as previously mentioned): *In Psychology, the tendency to attribute to others unacceptable impulses and traits that are present in one self. In extreme cases it may be pathological in nature, though generally it is one of the normal defence mechanisms;*

(3) **RATIONALIZATION***: A defence mechanism whereby the individual justifies his or her behavior by imposing on it a plausible rational explanation;*

(4) **REGRESSION***: A defence mechanism whereby an individual responds to stresses such as fear, frustration, or isolation, by reverting to behavior characteristic of a less complex, more primitive and impulsive stage of development. In psychoanalytic theory, the regression is either to an earlier state of libidinal interest and sexual organization or to an earlier stage of ego development. In the former, the person regresses from adult genitality to earlier (pre-genital) oral or anal sexual interest. In the latter, the person deals with the danger threatening him or her by behaving in a more childlike or generally primitive way* (Bullock et al, 1997);

(5) **DENIAL:** *A defence mechanism whereby one argues against an anxiety provoking stimuli by stating that it does not exist;*

(6) **DISPLACEMENT:**   A defence mechanism whereby a person takes out their impulses on a less threatening target;

(7) **INTELLECTUALIZATION:**   A defence mechanism where an individual avoids unacceptable or painful emotions by focusing on intellectual aspects of a situation;

(8) **REPRESSION:**   As previously mentioned, a defence mechanism whereby a person forgets an event by pulling it into the unconscious;

(9) **SUBLIMATION:**   A defence mechanism whereby an individual acts out unacceptable impulses in a socially acceptable way; and

(10) **SUPPRESSION:**   A defence mechanism whereby a person tries to forget something by pushing it into the unconscious (www.allpsych.com/psychology101/defenses.html, 2004).

Most of them are unsuccessful defences, that is, they do not succeed in getting rid of the dangerous impulse. Ego defence mechanisms are not necessarily unhealthy. Rather, the lack of such defences, or the inability to use them effectively, can lead to problems in life. However, we sometimes use these defence mechanisms at the wrong time or overuse them, which can be equally destructive (www.allpsych.com/psychology101, 2004).

Some symptoms of mental illness, such as irritability and aggression (as part of the 'manic' phase of bipolar disorder, for example), become inappropriately acted out when defence mechanisms like *projection* and *displacement* become extreme. As previously noted, the primitive tensions and needs if the *id* demand discharge, for example, by aggression against threats; in this case, perceived threats or when such threats do not exist. The mechanism to keep aggression in check, especially when a person may actually be *paranoid*, is weak, and this leads to *displacement* and *projection* to excess (as a defence mechanism) as the *ego* feels threatened by *false* impulses from the *id* (unconscious). Paranoia is discussed further in *PART III*.

According to Jeremy Griffith, in his book entitled *"Beyond the Human Condition"*:

> *Kept in the dark about what was going on, children have been left with no alternative but to block out pain which their parent's world of upset caused them. The most destructive element of the human condition was the silence and denial we had to practice. Unable to explain (defend) our upset state, we can't acknowledge its existence. Since upset first appeared, each new generation has had to learn to <u>repress</u> its true self and adopt prevailing levels of evasion, denial and silence. As this pattern is broken we will be able to speak the truth.*

> *The critical psychological point in our lives came when we resigned ourselves to 'reality'. We were born in to the world expecting it to be ideal and still like it was before upset appeared, only to discover it wasn't* (Griffith, 1991).

Griffith also stated that the most effective way to preserve the *soul* is not to let it go under in the first place.

The Seen But Forgotten

In the book "Destructive Emotions: A Dialogue with the Dalai Lama (and) Narrated by Daniel Goleman", it states in regards to the 'nature versus nurture' argument:

> *One of the most important human qualities may be our ability to regulate emotion- and here the frontal lobes appear to play a key role* [according to recent studies]. *One of the most exciting discoveries in neuroscience over the last ten years is that those areas of the brain-*
> *the frontal lobes, the amygdala, and the hippocampus, change in response to experience. These are the parts of the brain dramatically affected by the emotional environment in which we are raised and by repeated experience. This theme of how experience changes the brain- "neural plasticity"- is a central thread in further research and discussion* (Goleman, 2003, *'The Neuroscience of Emotion'*, p189).

This is some evidence, therefore, that environmental factors could also contribute much more towards a person developing a mental illness than has been more commonly acknowledged.

According to Goleman, what is particularly exciting about these findings is that the impact of environment on brain development has been traced down to the level of actual *gene expression*. This has only, so far, been done in animals, but it could apply to humans also. The other great finding in neuroscience is the fact that it has now been demonstrated in humans that new neurons do grow throughout the entire lifespan. Given this finding, it suggests then that it is possible also for one to recover from a mental illness over time, and that this finding offers great hope and benefits for people with mental illness. It also reinforces the fact that it is far more logical to only use psychotropic pharmaceutical drug therapy on a short-term basis, during crisis states of mind, because side effects and medical complications from some drugs can lead to premature death or suicides. This is discussed further in *PART VII-Medication Therapy: (The Dangers)*.

PART III

PARANOIA

Paranoia in the schizophreniform spectrum and other types of mental illness (such as bipolar disorder) can develop when susceptible or overly sensitive, or even damaged, individuals who lack a healthy sense of self worth unconsciously project onto others the way that they feel about themselves in order to blame others for their low self-esteem (Rose (ed), 1998). As explained in *Part II* (*The Big Picture: Some Possible Causes of Mental Illness*), this is not a conscious process, but it feels better for the person to attribute blame to others, instead of accepting painful acknowledgement that the feelings are arising from within the person. When the process of projection becomes pathological in such extreme cases resulting in the development of paranoia, this can lead to all sorts of disturbing thoughts and behaviors which to observers can also be frightening and difficult to understand.

A person who is paranoid (in the extreme) can, for example, start to believe that others are talking about them, staring at them, or even plotting to kill them. It is an extremely terrifying state of mind akin to 'a figment of the imagination', which is very hard to break free from when the sufferer is unwell without professional help, careful use of psychotropic medication, counseling, care and the development of good insight.

It should be said, however, that as thoughts about what other people are perceived to be saying about someone with paranoia worsen, the person can become so insecure that they may talk to themselves in many different manners, for example, hurtfully, encouragingly, grandiosely, biblically et cetera. This is sometimes due to the fact that, perhaps, the person has lost the ability to voice their opinions and believe in themselves and see their beliefs as meaningful. The paradox here is: people do sometimes talk about one another, and sometimes spitefully in an attempt to make someone feel left out. Thus, in an acutely sensitive or vulnerable individual, this can compound any tendency they may have towards developing paranoid thoughts and feelings.

In addition, a sensitive person can often be highly intuitive and this can be channeled to not so sensitive people, making them feel uncomfortable, so they set about the process of alienation of others or carrying out unconscious emotional abuse. The 'pre-schizophrenic' (sensitive) person does not imagine being treated differently. This can sometimes happen simply because they do not fit in, currently, in our society. The real trouble occurs when such a 'pre-schizophrenic' person allows this to get the better of them, due to low self-esteem and the absence of 'mirroring' from others so that they can actually have an understanding of themselves, and their gifts or differences from the 'norm'. This can then turn into self-loathing or self-torment, and a feeling that the world is against them. This, in turn, can only get worse the more the person does not seek (or cannot find) like-minded, sensitive, or perhaps highly artistic people, to help validate their feelings and views about the world they live in (Jacqueline Musgrave, 2005).

Of utmost importance for many sensitive individuals is to remember to have the ability to believe in themselves, regardless to whether or not they 'fit in' in our current society, and to keep searching for company and friends, and a sense of purpose.

The Seen But Forgotten

The thoughts and feelings that come with real paranoia can be so painful and disturbing to the person with a mental illness, such as schizophrenia, that the person may attempt to hurt themselves or others, in an attempt to escape the dreadful pain which they are experiencing. The sufferer is usually actually only a danger to himself (or herself), and not so much to others as many people tend to commonly believe.

Support from family, relatives and friends, and understanding from society as a whole, is very important for a paranoid person. Also, of course, help is needed from mental health professionals who can offer therapy to help build one's self-esteem, relieve stress and prescribe an appropriate medication if necessary. As the currently administered medications have their own shortfalls, they should only be used at lower doses for as minimal period of time as possible. The use of medication here has its place in some cases, whilst other options are not yet being explored by psychiatry and drug companies in relation to research being redirected in to naturopathic or homeopathic, or more 'natural' remedies. Modern chemical drugs should never be seen as a long-term solution, due to the adverse outcomes that they can produce for many people to whom they are given.

It is, somewhat understandably, difficult for the majority to understand the struggle of individuals with a mental illness in trying to create a life in a world which is built on a system of acceptance. In the positive light, however, this situation presents a challenge and an opportunity for the 'odd ball' to try to help make others aware, the general public or ordinary persons who accept too much things as they are, and are cut off from creative or other pursuits. The 'normal' person seeks security and comfort, and human feelings are not as important to them as their own security. Therefore, how can we expect the average person to have the level of compassion that is needed for those who suffer with a mental illness? This is where people and society as a whole must broaden their minds.

To reinforce the feeling, in some states of paranoia, that others are noticing a person, making it 'feel' as though others are staring or glaring at them, or talking about them, because they really do look so distressed or worried, people do in fact look at them and can ask themselves "I wonder what is wrong?" with him or her. This just compounds the situation. Delusions can also develop in more extreme paranoid states about being persecuted. For example, often depending on one's belief system, they can take on a 'messiahanic complex', perhaps in an attempt to explain to themselves why it is happening. The person may think 'I am Jesus Christ if I am suffering like this'. Or, the person may be in two minds about what is happening, at the feeling level. The sufferer may believe that the 'Devil' is responsible where this notion is part of a religious belief or preoccupation. At the time of having such feelings and thoughts, it is extremely difficult for a paranoid person to see that, as well as the underlying chemical or electrical imbalance in one's brain, due to whatever cause, we can also actually create our own 'demons', and that the mind is a very powerful thing. Paranoia is a state of mind, and can be a very frightening and tormenting one.

Once a person, who has experienced true paranoia, remembers and understands that he or she was paranoid, they can then try to recognize early warning signs; such as feeling mildly suspicious of others for no valid reason, or having a fleeting uncomfortable sense that people are talking about them in a nasty way, also for no good reason. With this insight, they could help ward off another full-blown episode which could occur by getting prompt help from their general practitioner, case manager or psychiatrist, as well as from any relatives or friends who could provide support. In the meantime, encouraging the person to try to reality test and challenge paranoid thoughts; write down or say out loud positive affirmations about themselves; or do anything positive to help build self-esteem or a fragile hurt state; these techniques can assist in lessening the severity of a possible paranoid episode.

PART IV

DELUSIONS

Delusions are very common in some forms of mental illness, for example in psychotic disorders like schizophrenia and bipolar disorder. A delusion is defined as a belief, or set of beliefs, often 'bizarre' and which are considered to have no basis in 'reality', yet which are often held as being true with real conviction by someone, despite evidence presented to the contrary. A belief is considered a delusion especially so where modern psychiatric associations and the average member of the public considers someone else's ideas or beliefs as not possible.

However, in some instances where a belief based on an experience is regarded as 'delusional', yet real sometimes, this is where society and psychiatrists need to be more open-minded. For example, in regards to some people's real psychic talents and abilities, and the real instances of extrasensory perception, these gifts and abilities are often negated by doubting and tutonic-thinking medical persons, who rely solely and purely on proof of everything via scientific and objective rules, and imply 'magical thinking' by the person in all cases. In these types of classifications of what is 'delusional', care needs to be taken in labeling a person who may really be a bit different or have outside of the 'norm' interests and talents. Here is where the danger lies in psychiatrists having too much power to be able to too easily label, misdiagnose and forcibly treat an otherwise very sane person.

On the other hand, of course, true delusional-thinking does happen. For example, many individuals who are experiencing extreme lack of self-worth, upset or abusive situations, and become mentally unwell, can and do conjure up inside their minds all sorts of 'fantasies' in an attempt to cope at times. Sometimes, this is to unconsciously protect their deep-seated hurt, and/or fragile sense of self-esteem. Or, it can happen when they are over-compensating with their ideas, identity, talents, and abilities, in an attempt to relieve the real pain which they are feeling. For example, this can happen in those with an underlying major depressive illness, or even a severe reactive depression from an intolerable life situation or event.

With respect to the illness known as 'bipolar disorder', people diagnosed with this condition can be in a 'mixed state", which is when the person is manic or 'hypomanic', yet feels 'bad' (dysphoric) or depressed at the same time. Here, often the person can actually start to think and believe that they are divinely chosen, extra special, or are another past or present famous person, whom obviously they are not. This can be attributed to being a kind of 'escape' in an attempt to regain some sense of self-worth where trauma has been suffered, such as sexual abuse as a child, for which proper counseling has not been thoroughly explored.

In regards to the mental illness labeled as 'schizophrenia', delusions can also develop. For example, they can occur where the sufferer can start to develop 'ideas of reference'; such as believing that characters in programs on the television are their family, or musicians singing their songs on the radio are directly speaking to them or about them or people they know. This is, once again, an unconscious escape, in an attempt to feel special or loved in extreme painful psychological states of upset or hurt. It is especially so where loneliness or social isolation compounds the situation, or when the sufferer has been through a major and severe stress or trauma at some time during their life and was unable to get the right help at the time. It is also especially so when the stress has occurred over a prolonged period of time. Ideas of reference can also occur just after a major upset which was so severe as to trigger a 'psychosis' in an acutely sensitive person.

These 'states of mind' can be so real or terrifying to the sufferer that they can become angry, abusive, confused, or so scared that suicide may be attempted. And, hallucinations, such as, auditory, tactile or visual in nature can make it even worse. Here, seeking prompt professional care and advice can help the person to settle a bit, to try to develop some insight and challenge some of their thoughts, and help to encourage the person to develop 'cognitive thinking strategies' to assist with performing reality checks. This is necessary to help the person experiencing these symptoms in combination with their doctor prescribing lower doses of appropriate medication which suits best a particular person's physiology. Regrettably, there is still no existent of any better and safer medications or treatments.

It can be with delusional thinking, sometimes, what one is telling oneself. Educational cognitive therapy needs to be carried out in a safe and non-threatening environment, in order to help people who do develop delusions to become grounded again. Here is where fully-trained and qualified psychologists can help on a one-to-one basis to provide counseling and therapy, and help teach people with mental illness about their condition and how to try to stay in touch with truth. The term 'reality' is not used here as it is too indefinable to be applicable, given the variations in the nature of different people's different beliefs, cultures and experiences.

Sometimes, a person who has a mental illness can become so exhausted with trying to cope with their condition on a continual basis that they can lose their resolve or their ability to deal with their symptoms. At the moment, this is especially so when there has been little or no treatment carried out to attempt to get to the root cause of one's illness, and the person has received little real therapy to promote healing and recovery. This is especially so where doctors are focusing too much on treating the symptoms only. Healing and recovery are not abstract concepts with any real possibility. It is about time that modern medicine focused more on this and moved aside somewhat to allow psychologists to carry out more work with people diagnosed with mental illness.

For people trying to cope with their mental disorder, becoming tired and occasionally relapsing, this is something that normal, healthy people tend to take for granted. That is, for example, where normal people do not have to cope with 'hearing voices' or sometimes frightening visual hallucinations or delusions. Most 'healthy' people in society also do not seem to have as much physical and emotional sensitivity as those who become unwell or delusional. This is why it is so important for the person, who is unwell, as part of their journey of recovery, or in trying to recover, to be able to say to themselves: "I am just going to be who I am", and try to relax and trust in the process. This is not an easy thing to do, by any means. And, obviously, there are many hurdles to overcome along the way.

PART V

DEPRESSION

Depression is one of the most common problems that many people today will experience in modern society. According to recent figures, around 20 per cent of adults, world wide, will experience an episode of depression serious enough to warrant professional help.

Depression is not just any bad or upsetting feeling. For example, depression is not where a person feels anxious, although it is common that depressed individuals frequently feel anxious when they are depressed. Some of the characteristics of a depressive illness are defined by psychiatry as:-

- ➢ Dysphoria, or feeling 'bad' most of the time;
- ➢ A low level of activity or a lack of motivation;
- ➢ Problems with interacting with other people;
- ➢ Feelings of worthlessness and inadequacy;
- ➢ Feelings of guilt or that one deserves to be punished for their 'badness';
- ➢ Feeling burdened;
- ➢ Difficulty concentrating; and
- ➢ Physical problems, such as a lack of energy, sleep disturbances, poor appetite, and increased frequency of headaches, stomachaches and intestinal difficulties
  (Lewinsohn et al, 1986).

Emotions such as guilt and worthlessness, associated with depression, are very debilitating and hard to bear. This can be compounded by a fear of not being understood, or of being misjudged by others, even in some cases by nursing staff in the hospital setting.

Psychological counseling is, obviously, necessary for a depressed person, for them to be able to see that they are not unwell because they are *weak or not trying*. It can be a vicious cycle when a person is depressed if they blame themselves or are given a hard time by others. The chief goal of therapy here is to try to relieve such stress and anxiety and promote personal growth, and to help the person avoid such self-destructive ways of thinking (which are part of the illness) to avoid further chaos and rifts in mental life.

Strategies for all sufferers of clinical depression to increase self-esteem (and self-worth) are very important for understanding and recovery, in combination with the right medication, and to realize that there is 'light at the end of the tunnel'. With improved self-esteem will come a lessening of feelings of depression and anxiety, and a quicker recovery from depressive illness. This is where as much help as possible is necessary from family, friends, carers and mental health professionals, in order for people generally to better understand just how frightening and painful it can be for a person who is suffering with depression. Even when insight is reasonable and reality checks are possible, it is still very frightening, as the person knows here that they are not fully in control of their thoughts and feelings. Without prompt medical intervention and psychological counseling here, the level of suffering for a person's mind and body when they are clinically depressed can be extremely acute, serious enough to lead to them taking their own life. Alternately, when help is sought and provided, depression is a very treatable illness and good recovery rates occur.

As well as taking some medication, when symptoms are so acute as to be life-threatening, it is also important for a person who is severely depressed to make some small efforts to overcome the depression as they start to feel better from the effects of taking the right anti-depressant drug. Cognitive behavioral therapy taught by psychologists and psychiatrists can be very helpful in helping the person avoid cognitive distortions in their thinking, such as, 'all-or-nothing thinking'; 'overgeneralizations'; and 'black and white thinking'. With consistent efforts can come small rewards, and with this can come some hope and growth in one's life and their journey along the road to recovery.

One can also change one's 'world' by changing one's beliefs, if the belief or set of beliefs is creating turmoil and intense upset. For example, excessive and inappropriate guilt feelings, perhaps brought on by extremist views which have been imposed on someone who was vulnerable – this has happened to mankind throughout our history – can be relieved in the person by them doing some personal soul-searching to try to work out and decide what they prefer to believe without fear of recrimination or punishment. Throughout the generations, often some of the different religions which have been man-made have attempted to control people and instill fear and guilt into people. In some cases, the more sensitive and vulnerable individuals who are subject to this type of indoctrination can become confused, very scrupulous and as a result, become mentally unwell. As this begins to happen less, people will be able to speak more freely, with less guilt, fear and scruples, and the development and instance of depression in more vulnerable individuals will become less.

Lewinsohn et al reported that not everyone experiences depression in the same way. Some people will feel guilty and have trouble sleeping and eating when depressed; others will isolate themselves and feel lonely and friendless; still others will cry often and give up their usual pleasant activities (Lewinsohn et al, 1986).

Lewinsohm et al also noted that:

Every depressed person has a unique set of specific problems (Lewinsohn et al, 1986).

The authors considered the following factors in a *Self-Assessment in Taking Stock of Your Problems*, by one creating a plan to overcome depression, including considering:

- **Relaxation**
- **Pleasant activities**
- **Problems with people**
- **Troublesome thoughts**
- **Approaching your problems constructively**
- **Self-control problems**

(Lewinsohn et al, 1986)

Additional factors which can help reduce the acuteness of depression in someone who is unwell are:

- Physical exercise
- A healthy diet
- Setting small goals
- Getting adequate and restful sleep
- Avoiding alcohol and illicit drugs
- Journaling feelings and thoughts

Depression can often result from unresolved, bottled up anger and grief; where one has not been able to successfully let go of hurt and past trauma. This lack of being able to 'let go' can be unhealthy and affect a person's thoughts, feelings and state of mind. In addition, where a person has a lack of loving relationships and experiences loneliness, and little sense of purpose, even meaning in their life; this can increase any tendencies that a person has in experiencing depression. Here is where therapy with trained counselors and psychologists can also assist in helping someone in this type of situation the skills necessary for them to help themselves and try to overcome their depression. With every little success, this only serves to breed more success.

In Melody Beattie's book, *The Language of Letting Go*, she recommends that:

Sometimes, even if we don't feel like we have let go or can let go, we can "act as if" we have, and that will help bring about the letting go we desire. You don't have to give up your power to problems. You can take your focus off your problem and direct it to your life, trusting that doing so will bring you closer to a solution (Beattie, 1990).

A meditation which Beattie suggests; one that someone can use in attempting to let go of a problem or bothersome thoughts is:

Today, I will go on living my life and tending to my routine. I will decide, as often as I need to, to stop obsessing about whatever is bothering me. If I don't feel like letting go of a particular thing, I will "act as if" I have let go of it until my feelings match my behavior (Beattie, 1990).

Apart from relying solely on medication as a treatment for some forms of clinical depression, it is also important for the depressed person to think about constructive ways of 'letting go' of problems, and practicing ways to let go of anger, hurt, frustration, and even fear. This can help in reducing the severity of the suffering experienced when one is feeling depressed, or in the midst of a full blown major depressive disorder.

PART VI

SCHIZOPHRENIA: AN INNER HELL AND STATE OF MIND

'Schizophrenia', a term derived from the Greek meaning 'split mind', is an illness and state of mind which can be experienced as a state of self-torment. Such a state of mind can be brought on by an excessive tendency in a person to be fearful and when they may have a lack of 'knowing', and lack trust. For example, when a person experiences, as we all do at times, *'a fear of the unknown'*, and lacks the necessary trust in others and the normal flow of things and progression of life, this can create in some instances extremely excessive levels of *anxiety*. In addition, the fears and anxiety experienced by the sufferers of schizophrenia can be exacerbated by intense and out-of-proportion feelings of hurt in acutely sensitive, young individuals, as a result of real cruelty inflicted by others, and, in some cases, even imagined abuse. People with schizophrenia do tend to be overly sensitive to criticism and/or even bad treatment from others, and tend to take 'things to heart' a lot more so than others. Young people who break down and develop schizophrenia also seem to be the more soft, sensitive, creative and artistic souls of our world, who have suffered negligence or abuse, and can see, and get terribly upset about, some of the cruelties and injustices that continue to occur in the world. This also creates fear in their psyches.

The propensity to tap into the states of fear by some people with schizophrenia seems to be exacerbated or heightened as a result of the sufferer focusing too much on the polarization of beliefs in society, all over the world, and their (and our) tendency to assume that the other party is wrong, or even 'evil'. Opposing sides with their differing experiences and views assumes that the other is involved in a conspiracy of some kind. One does not have to suffer from schizophrenia to do this though. However, people with schizophrenia seem to be more vulnerable to feelings of more intense fear and anxiety, to the point of becoming paranoid and making up elaborate conspiracy theories, such as the C.I.A. is after them, which are *not* true, but delusional. These kinds of ideas and theories seem to satisfy some sort of overly self-centered agenda. By 'self-centered', this is not necessarily equated with selfishness or manipulative ness, but rather a sense or feeling within the sufferer that they are extra special, in an attempt to overcompensate and relieve bad feelings of fear and anxiety, and even depression. People with schizophrenia may not be extra special, but they are special by the fact that they can possess great artistic talent, and can hallucinate imaginary friends (or the 'spaceship') to talk to, to comfort them when they become insular. However, having visual or auditory hallucinations of imaginary enemies is often very tormenting for sufferers and is why help is necessary to try to stop this happening for them.

Sometimes, those people who have schizophrenia tend to want, more so than others, for the world to be *perfect* because they often when they are young cannot cope with the way the world actually is. Sometimes they cannot face reality, or so-called 'reality', which is often described as an *illusion* in the spiritual or metaphysical sense*.

*Metaphysics is the study of the philosophy of being and truth. The concept of illusions versus reality is too broad a concept to discuss here and goes beyond the purpose of this book.

The Seen But Forgotten

As a consequence, they can decide to unconsciously escape and become out of touch with 'reality', usually due to confusion and excessive fear, which is somehow also related to an underlying chemical imbalance of neurotransmitters in the 'schizophrenic' brain, and which is not yet fully understood. However, it has been noted that many special and sensitive people who develop schizophrenia come from families brought up under some religions, extreme discipline and extremely upsetting and dysfunctional family environments, with huge guilt-based beliefs, and even child abuse, such as violent, dictatorial and over-controlling parenting.

The type of schizophrenia induced by fearful thinking, leading to paranoia, insularism, sometimes panic, and a loss of the connection with the inner self, can lead to an unintentional, self-induced 'hellish' state of mind. At this time, the sufferer cannot see any way to process their conflicting thoughts and emotions, and incoming sensory information, and so, they become 'split' in their mind, creating all sorts of frightening thoughts, feelings, sometimes hallucinations, and behaviors. When this happens, that is, when anger and intense fear arise, it is so important for the person experiencing these symptoms, to try to attempt to be mindful, take a step back if possible, and be helped to recognize that these thoughts and feelings are states of mind and symptoms of the illness.

Of course, over time, it would take a lot of learning and practice for one to become adept in doing this. In addition, concentrating on proper breathing, calm meditation on some different questions or problems done in a positive way, can help still the mind and allow thoughts and feelings to make better sense. Not everybody suffering from a schizophrenic state of mind is able to do this, especially during a first episode of psychosis, without a lot of help and support, and some psychotropic medication. Many people with schizophrenia would also be helped by being able to process, come to terms with, and let go of past traumas, as well as being able to seek out and have positive friendships with other like-minded individuals. This could then help them to be able to take on board more positive messages, to help counteract the negativity, doubts and fears, where some *balance* indicators, reassurance and understanding from others is required.

Some young people with schizophrenia also tend to take 'the problems of the world', so to speak, on to their shoulders; even to the extent of thinking that it is up to them to fix things all by themselves. In the extreme, some even tend to do this to the extent where they blame themselves for catastrophies, such as a natural disaster or war in some part of the world, for which, obviously, they had no part to play in whatsoever. Here, they exhibit an underlying or inherent tendency of being extremely sensitive to unfortunate and cruel happenings in life. This type of thinking can induce intense and painful, inappropriate feelings of guilt. This can place the sufferer under enormous pressure and tension, which is totally incongruous to what, is true. Such guilt can also lead to shame, which if progresses to a toxic degree, can physically and emotionally paralyse such a sensitive individual. The person can then behave and act in such a way which appears strange to others. For example, the 'stilted wooden gait', as observed by clinicians, where the sufferer appears very stiff and stilted in their motor functions, as well as very emotionally stressed.

The sufferer can also become so emotionally crippled or confused enough to not know *who they are.* As a result, they lose their natural vivacity and can appear distracted. This includes where they may also not know what they want to do in life or what to 'become' in order to gain acceptance, and a sense of well being and purpose in life. This can happen due to being placed in double bind situations or scenarios of extreme emotional blackmail by parents when young, and by the sort of parent who decides to impose their will on their children's lives. They have not been allowed to follow their own basic healthy life instincts, drives and ambitions, and are sometimes controlled to the extent that their natural inherent talents and abilities are stifled to the point of mental breakdown; and, in some cases, having a 'death wish'. In such a state, naturally, this robs the child of drive and motivation, as commonly observed by other normal members of society, including family, peers and friends. This only further serves to alienate them from ordinary or everyday life. Unfortunately, they can be misjudged by the layperson as being weak, lazy or apathetic; when what the person with schizophrenia really needs to be able to do (and be helped to do) is to get rid of the false guilt and shame which is binding them. Also, they need to be helped to try to see what is real: that is, that some unfortunate and tragic situations are an inevitable and real part of life (for reasons we do not yet fully understand). They need to be helped to realize that these events are out of their direct control or any one person's control.

Some of the scenarios which upset many are what man inflicts on man. The human race is still evolving out of the animal stage, and sensitive people with schizophrenia do tend to be very loving and sensitive to the injustices of the world, and more so to their own traumas which they have experienced. Wishful thinking combined with a desire to escape, can lead to a 'flight from reality' for people susceptible to psychosis in schizophrenia.

Some young and sensitive people with schizophrenia would like to be able to save the world. However, obviously, no single person is, or can be, the 'centre of the Universe', as some sufferers of schizophrenia can sometimes tend to think or feel, or simply *wish* to be at times. Here, it would also be important for one to try to achieve some balance in their thinking and in how they perceive the world. As previously mentioned elsewhere in this book, anyone can change their world by *changing their beliefs*. It is not so much about behavior modification as it is about thoughts and beliefs modification in attempting to be who you really are. Each of us can only try to do our best by contributing what we can, in a co-operative, positive and loving fashion, and recognize that nobody and nothing in life is, or was meant to be, perfect, or even easy. No single person in life is perfect, and our life experiences are not always positive, as this would mean that we would never be able to make mistakes from which to *learn* things. And, of course, there are many lessons for us all to learn in life. Otherwise, we would all be like robots, and life itself would have no real point.

In some people who have schizophrenia, who may have very altruistic intentions for their life, it is important for them to also be able to face the fact that even though life *is* hard, it can also bring many rewards and much happiness. However, this is not to say that we are or were meant to continue to develop through suffering. We can also develop through and strive for peace and harmony, whilst at the same time finding it challenging to do this. The universal hope for a better world or the "Second Coming" has been defined as:

when each person realizes that they are involved in saving humanity; and when each one of us comes to our true potential (Berther, April 2007).

The Seen But Forgotten

Being able to recognize that life is hard, as, of course, many people realize, some sufferers of schizophrenia may not be able to accept it fully? Given this point, with respect to the current medical treatments for schizophrenia, the use of (still at the present time, dangerous) drugs, does play a role in attempting to relieve and control the often distressing symptoms of psychosis and depression. The modern anti-psychotic drugs are, though, fraught with their own problems and can lead to physical health complications. For example, many can cause obesity, diabetes, heart disease and resultant complications leading to premature death. And, in some cases, some of the physical drug side effects of most anti-psychotic drugs, such as akathisia and tardive dyskinesia, can be as torturous and painful as to cause the person suffering with these drug-induced conditions to try to kill themselves. In many cases, the sufferer succeeds in their suicide attempt. Therefore, the current medical drug treatments, often still forced on already suffering people, are still very primitive and cruel, reminiscent of the trial and error and experimentation days of not so long ago, where frontal lobotomies, ice cube shock treatment, deep sleep therapy and other horrors were inflicted on people with mental illness; and where so many people died. This was covered-up by governments, psychiatrists and the institutions of the day. However, some of the stories related to these real events are now being told and more information is becoming available.

Victoria Musgrave

PART VII

MEDICATION THERAPY: (THE DANGERS)

Neuroscientists use the term 'working memory' for the capacity of attention that holds in mind the facts essential for completing a given task or solving a problem (Goleman, 1996). The use of prolonged and heavy doses of major tranquilizers (or 'anti-psychotic' medications) and the over-use of minor tranquilizers (the benzodiazepine group of drugs) can 'anaesthetize' the emotions, cause over-sedation, and thus interfere with one's working memory to the extent that it becomes extremely difficult for the person taking these drugs to take part in any cognitive therapy.

If the person is not able to take part in some psychological therapy to help to get to the root cause of their problems, how are they expected to truly recover well and eventually wean off the medication where possible? The medications used for all sorts of mental illnesses, including for anxiety disorders and psychotic disorders are merely a 'band aid' approach to treating the illness. Apart from this, eventually, due to their extremely toxic chemical nature and the fact that they are poisonous to the body and brain, they can lead to premature death from medical complications such as weight gain, heart disease and diabetes. This is not to mention some of the other more rapidly-occurring extra pyramidal side effects (such as akathisia and other dystonic reactions) after ingestion which can be extremely painful to the person taking them, sometimes, as previously mentioned, leading to suicide attempts. As explained in more detail in the *Introduction,* there can be many unwanted reactions and side effects of both antipsychotic medications and benzodiazepine drugs.

In addition, functioning well generally becomes very difficult and these individuals often appear bombed-out and 'zombie-like'. This also leads to suicide by some people from their sense of despair and knowing that this is 'as good as it gets'. Apart from other distressing extra pyramidal side effects of anti-psychotics, such as restlessness and uncontrollable abnormal movements, due to not being able to function normally as others do (and take for granted) this increases depression, lowers self-esteem and sense of meaning and purpose in life, and makes it very difficult for people on these drugs to ever experience any normality, including meaningful occupations or activities, such as employment.

An effective balance is required when it comes to prescribing therapeutic doses of currently-favored medications, until better ones are produced, in order to still allow the person taking them to function to their best and be able to have some quality of life. Until recovery is helped along via psychological counseling methods and cognitive work, with the aim of taking the person off medication to help avoid premature death, current pharmaceutical drugs should only be used with great caution. If they do ease suffering (not increase it), are not seen as a something that a person who has a mental illness needs to take for the rest of their life, and as there is nothing else yet which doctors can prescribe which could be safer, there is no other real option at present. Unfortunately, modern psychiatry has no real basis in medicine and has lost its original intention, that is, from the 'Greek' meaning: 'soul healing'. Today, psychiatry, especially in the public health system, seems to only rely on so-called 'observations' and symptomatology, without considering the root cause/s and an individual's real needs, including some basics; such as a healthy diet, appropriate accommodation and social environments, enough exercise and meaningful relationships, employment or other activities.

There is no doubt that for some people with mental illness who do not seem to have as many chemical and physical sensitivities as others, taking medication which does help them in the short term; here it can and does play an important role in reducing symptoms and giving good relief. However, over time, long term problems can arise which can target this group and lead to early death from physical illnesses caused by taking the drugs. This is mainly from the medical complications associated with weight gain, as mentioned previously. Since chemical therapy has been introduced, trialed and prescribed, side effects have been shown to be extremely bothersome for most people though. This has led to international drug companies furthering their research to try to produce 'better' medications, which have fewer side effects and are superior in controlling symptoms. It remains to be seen if this is the way to go in providing treatments for mental illnesses, or even a cure for some.

For some people, though, certain medications, prescribed 'Willy nilly', particularly with the use of anti-psychotics and certain antidepressants, can lead to a worsening of, or even mimic, the illness for which it was originally prescribed. This fact is often negated by the drug companies and psychiatrists because they do not want to admit that some of their ideas and methods could be wrong; and because this would mean that they would lose a lot of money, and have to actually prove that mental illness can be scientifically explained as being caused by a 'chemical imbalance'. This theory has been debunked by some physicians around the world. There has been no blood test, or other test, so far yet which can be done to show such a chemical imbalance, purported to be the cause of a person's mental 'disorder'. In addition, psychiatry just keeps on making up more and more (even bigger and better) labels for a myriad of new so-called illnesses and 'disorders', for which the research is being partly funded by drug companies. This would appear to be a conflict of interest; or vested interests.

Each person's physiology is different from another's, and this needs to be taken into account whilst modern pharmaceutical drugs continue to be administered – until more suitable treatments are considered by putting more funding and research into less chemically-based medications, and naturopathic and homeopathic medicines are developed for the treatment of mental illness. Another consideration would be to look into research in Chinese herbal medicine and acupuncture, as a safer alternative in treating mental illness. The toxic approach to modern psychiatry constitutes an overhaul of their and the drug companies' theories in order to help design much more suitable and successful treatments and therapies for people with mental illness.

Psychiatry, therapy, and even mental health hospitals do have a place in our society where vulnerable and unwell individuals can find it too hard to cope with life at times, and voluntarily agree to have some 'time out'. However, the history, and even with respect to what still happens today, and the practice of psychiatry in the public institutions and hospitals has been experimental and cruel, and there is a great need for much improvement in order for people with mental illness to be treated with more dignity and respect and not have to suffer as much as they have and still do. In some developed countries, such as the United Kingdom and America, the practice of psychiatry is seen by some as an agent of social repression, in league with society and the family at large in putting pressure on non-conforming individuals. This view could be considered extreme, as it seems to imply that mental illness does not really exist? As previously noted, this is not the subject of argument put forward here. Mental illness does exist. However, it is the concern about the treatments for it which are the issues considered in this book. Nevertheless, many psychiatrists and families have indeed made 'scape goats' out of 'non-conforming' individuals and placed them in institutions as part of a cover-up, or simply to shut up a family member who is reeling against abuse and victimization.

Psychiatry has come some way since the 1980's, but it has not yet come far enough where some cruel practices are still employed, such as holding people down and injecting them with an antipsychotic medication. Before the introduction of pharmaceutical drugs, during the even more experimental times of the late 1800's and mid 1900's in mental institutions, there were performed hundreds of leucotomies, frontal lobotomies, hysterectomies, electric shock treatments without anesthetic, and insulin shock treatments. Not to mention the experiments by a psychiatrist during the 1980's at Chelmsford Private Hospital (established in 1963 in Sydney, New South Wales), where many people died under his 'deep sleep' treatments; and the verbal and physical abuse and restrictions on liberty that patients were subjected to in Ward 10B in Townsville (North Queensland) during the 1970's and 1980's, as part of a so-called 'therapeutic environment'. In 'Wolston Park' (now called 'The Park', Queensland Centre for Mental Health Research, Education and Training) in Wacol (South East Queensland), which was established in 1865; one hundred and forty years ago; during the late 1960s, less than fifty per cent of patient's survived the first year of treatment, both male and female

(Campbell et al, 2008; Newsletter, the Schizophrenia Fellowship of Queensland Inc., 2007).

Some of the earlier anti-psychotic drugs (or 'typical' major tranquilizers), such as modecate, and haloperidol (a drug said to have been designed in Nazi Germany by their pharmaceutical scientists), which thankfully tend not to be used today, were also classics in causing unbearable physical side effects, like extreme restlessness and stiffness. Yet, the person was expected to and often forced to keep taking these drugs, despite the obvious severe physical pain they were experiencing. (The *Introduction* to this book explained in more depth the difficulties of taking and changing psychotropic medications, what some of the specific side effects are, and what they are named by the medical profession).

At present, because of the dangers of modern psychiatric practice and the fact that mental illness continues to be an issue in society; if society refuses to admit that we also need to broaden our minds and aim also at treating the causes of mental illness and attempt to remove the possible causes, the use of chemical therapy will, unfortunately, continue to be used. It will not be until more psychologists and counselors are trained and employed to help those who have mental illness; and more research is done into the possibilities of treating mental illness using more 'natural' substances; that current psychiatric practice can be modified and life-threatening chemical drug treatments can be abolished.

In 2000, the Australian Federal Government distributed an information brochure on the nationwide abuse of marijuana. However, this does not appear to have had any effect. In 1999, the Federal Police advised that they had no jurisdiction over the use of dangerous drugs in Queensland Health psychiatric institutions because the Queensland Government maintained that the drugs were legal and not banned substances. Therefore, when security personnel subdued patients for the nurses to inject dangerous drugs, the action was legal. In 1999 also, the Queensland Police Minister, Tony McGrady, assured Berther that Queensland police were training officers to be aware of their powers under the new Mental Health Act 2000.

Berther stated:

If I held somebody down and injected them with dangerous drugs, I would be charged with either grievous bodily harm or attempted manslaughter as applicable. Mental Health Act (MHA) 2000 allows nurses and security personnel to do so "without liability". The action is approved and ordered by psychiatric registrars and psychiatric consultants, and then condoned by nurse unit managers, assistant directors of nursing and directors of nursing, and finally by the Director of the Mental Health Unit (MHU); together with the administrator of the MHU.

MHA 2000 allows for patients to be placed in "seclusion". There are set processes directed by the Act. These processes are still ignored by Princess Alexandra Hospital Mental Health Unit nurses and doctors "without liability". Patients who "refuse" to take "dangerous drugs" are still beaten into submission by security personnel in PAH MHU (Berther, 2007).

The Mental Health Act 2000 absolves everybody from liability for anything under Section 536 and the sixth line of the introductory paragraph. MHA 2000 has provision for anybody to have any person committed to a psychiatric institution with no justification whatever; without sworn statements to a magistrate, and without any checks made by police or competent mental health workers. The police "assisting" the doctor and nurse do not even have to show the warrant. MHA 2000 puts the icing on the cake by stating on the sixth line: "the State" is not liable for any act committed. Section 536 absolves "any person" acting "with authority" from liability. The liability reverts to the "State".

Berther asked:

Was this Act really compiled by "barristers from Victoria" as I was led to believe by Queensland Health in 1999? It was going to be the "Utopian Act" in health care! Did the formulation of the new act really have input of consumers as I was assured?

Also according to Berther:

Take a look at the results of Mental Health Act 2000. Patients are still dying from the effects of psychiatric drugs, as well as from the traditional suicide method; which in many cases is probably induced by the effects of the modern hallucinatory psychotropic medication together with the "fat drugs" olanzapine, clozapine and risperidone (the death drugs).

Now is the time for a National Mental Health Act. A well presented document such as Mental Health Act (MHA) 1974/Mental Health Regulation (MHR) 1985 (without the provision of Section 69), which has checks and balances. One must follow "the rules", do the "paperwork", and consider the rights of "voluntary patients" to refuse medication and discharge themselves. MHA 2000 has no such provisions. The paperwork does not have to be completed. Warrants do not have to be shown to the patient. For example, a section states steps (1), (2),(3),(4),(5), and (6) must happen. But (7) states that the action is still legal if (4), (5), and (6) do not happen: NO LIABILITY AT ALL.

Queensland government advertisements promoting tolerance and understanding of mental health in the community are regular issues. Why not follow the same ethics inside the MHU's? Why employ thugs who masquerade as security officers? Why force patients to ingest the "death drugs"? Why employ psychiatric registrars who outdo Hans Christian Anderson in fabricating "fairy tales" which are then submitted to the Mental Health Tribunal? Why employ psychiatric consultants who cannot speak English prohibiting any communication with the patient? Why employ mental health directors whose apparent role is to "put out bushfires" and "cover-up illegal acts" by pretending that correct records have not been kept; apparently in collusion with "consumer representatives"?

Why change MHA 1974/MHR 1985 which was "the goods", and replace it with MHA 2000 thereby eliminating accountability, liability, morals and ethics? (Berther, 2007).

Victoria Musgrave

PART VIII

THE HOPE FOR RECOVERY

Mental illness or mental challenges are very common. They are more common than cancer, diabetes or heart disease. The question is: is there hope for recovery? Several studies have now shown that many people experiencing serious and persistent mental health problems can and do recover.

There is a certain amount of grief that can come from any type of illness, be it physical or mental. With respect to mental health issues, recovery is about one accepting that, for now, they have a mental illness and endeavoring to develop insight into their condition. Then, it becomes about trying to manage one's illness to the best of one's ability. Insight and good judgment needs to be there for a person to try to get the most out of life, and have the best possible quality of life despite having an illness. For example, if a person knows that they *are* manic (elevated in their mood), they need to know it, deal with it, get some help and still be surviving; at least until the manic episode subsides so that normality can be resumed again.

The journey of recovery is a process, not a destination or even a cure. The goal of recovery should be to move away from defining oneself by the label given by an illness or the symptoms one may experience. It should also be about regaining a sense of positive self-worth that enables a person to reestablish meaning in life.

Mental health recovery has been defined as:

The individual process of overcoming the negative impact of a psychiatric disability despite its continued presence (www.themainplace.org/).

In other words, recovery is the process by which an individual recovers their self-esteem, identity, self-worth, dreams, pride, choice, dignity and a meaningful life (The Main Place, Your Place to Recover, internet).

Patricia Deegan Ph.D., Director of Training, of the National Empowerment Center, has had first hand experience of mental illness. Her first steps of recovery, as defined by Anna Huskey (National Alliance for the Mentally Ill Santa Cruz County website) at the 'Partners in Recovery Adult System of Care Conference 2000', were strategies such as:

- *No illicit/street drugs or alcohol*
- *Be in a tolerant environment*
- *Have a relationship with people who care about you and you care about them*
- *Spirituality: finding meaning in your suffering*
- *Have a sense of purpose and direction*
- *Dare to have a dream*
- *Have routine*
- *Take a day at a time, an hour at a time, a minute at a time*
- *Study, learn and work*

(www.namiscc.org/newsletters, 2005).

Patricia Deegan, a clinical psychologist, has noted in some of her talks data from several longitudinal studies:

Long-term studies have consistently found that one half to two thirds of people diagnosed with mental illness go on to a significant or complete recovery. Data shows that even in the second or third decade a person can still go on to complete recovery. I believe you can be one of the ones to recover. I am here to support your journey of recovery.

According to Huskey, Deegan also stated that there is no way of knowing who will be the ones to recover. At the onset of the illness, recovery should not be ruled out as a possibility for anyone. Recovery, it was noted, is not something that we wait until later to talk about. By allowing the possibility of recovery, we can then enable the road to be made by traveling along it.

Deegan also pointed out that some people have found neuroleptic medications to be helpful. However, she stated that the story that does not get told is how many people get buried under medication. Deegan said:

There are legions of people who are drugged out of their gourd. I will ask for the rational use of medication. To use medicine along with self help strategies. Compliance is not the road to recovery. There needs to be room for the consumer to make mistakes. If a mistake is made we do not abandon clients to suffer the natural consequences of their choices. Change is inevitable, progress is optional.

In a *National Research Project for the Development of Recovery Facilitating System Performance Indicators,* regarding mental health recovery: *What Helps and What Hinders?* This study looked at consumer perspectives on what helps and what hinders recovery (www.namiscc.org, October 2002). The participating states were Arizona, Colorado, New York, Oklahoma, Rhode Island, South Carolina, Texas, Utah and Washington.

The five-person research team, each with significant recovery research experience, outlined at the outset of the study five important factors to recovery: *resources/basic needs, choices/self-determination, independence, interdependence/connective ness, and hope.* The study also extrapolated on the emergent themes of: *basic material resources, self/whole person, hope/ sense of meaning and purpose, social relationships, meaningful activities, peer support, formal services, and formal service staff.*

The study also pointed out that while recovery is a deeply personal journey, there are many commonalities in people's experiences and opinions:

Recovery is a product of dynamic interaction among characteristics of the individual, characteristics of the environment, and the characteristics of the exchange (www.namiscc.org, 2002).

Within this ecological context, basic material resources, a livable income, safe and decent housing, healthcare, transportation, a means of communication (for example, a telephone), move people towards recovery. It was found that poverty and a lack of basic resources undermine a sense of safety and hold people back in their recovery.

Along with basic material needs, it emerged also that:

People need opportunities and supports to engage in the responsibilities and benefits of citizenship, of membership to community. Recovery involves a social dimension, a core of active, interdependent social relationships being connected through families, friends, peers, neighbours, and colleagues in mutually supportive and beneficial ways. Social and personal isolation, poverty, emotional withdrawal, controlling relationships, poor social skills, immigrant status, emotionally disabling health and mental health conditions, past trauma, and social stigma impede the recovery journey (www.namiscc.org, 2002).

According to Doug Dornan, when considering the fullness of personhood and the self-agency dimension to recovery, the study researchers were struck by how much their findings related to a sought universal quality of life needs and desires. Participants' life journeys began prior to the onset of mental illness and continue after. It was found that *hope* advances many people's life journeys. Therefore, a *holistic* focus and positive attitude, beliefs and goals, on one's own part, on the part of families and careers, and in the media and broader community, can help to promote and move recovery forward.

Dornan also stated that:

Full citizenship expands beyond social relationships. Participants indicated that recovery is enhanced through engaging in meaningful activities that connect one to the community. Often this can be achieved through a meaningful job and career, which can provide a sense of identity and mastery. Participants also identified other options, such as advancing one's education, volunteering, engaging in group advocacy efforts, and/or being involved in program design and policy level decision-making. Participants report high rates of unemployment, underemployment, and exploitation. Training and education opportunities are lacking, benefits have employment disincentives, prejudice and discrimination hamper efforts, and individual wishes and decisions are disregarded.
(www.namiscc.org, 2002).

Overall, Dornan's study showed that 'personhood' serves as a central dimension to recovery. Participants talked about an internal 'sense of self', inner strivings and their 'whole being' (physical, emotional, mental, and spiritual) as being affected by, as well as affecting the recovery process.

As we saw in *PART II*, according to the theory surrounding 'neural-plasticity', new neurons in the brain do grow throughout our entire lifespan. One can retrain the brain by the way we think, and thus help to correct the underlying malfunction of cells and resultant chemical imbalance, which is a supposed partial cause of mental illness. Therefore, we cannot afford the luxury of negative thoughts all of the time. It is possible; and where cognitive behavioural therapy (CBT) would be useful; to train oneself out of 'negative thinking' (even paranoia). Negative thinking is common in mental illness, especially in clinical depression and schizophrenia. By increasing self-esteem through thinking more positive thoughts, we can help change, not only our thoughts and state of mind, but our behaviour too. Then, recovery becomes about growing as a person, 'letting go' of past trauma, and replacing unloving or negative thoughts with positive messages and more loving thoughts. There would be a shift in someone's perception in their life and of others, and maturity develops and healing takes place. This kind of *shift in perception* can produce miraculous results in the recovery process in people who have serious mental health issues and mental illness.

By one changing their thought processes consciously (with effort and practice), one can eventually recover from mental illness or mental health problems, even eventually come off medication over decent measures of time - to allow the receptors and neurons in the brain to return to normal as emotional healing takes place. All mental illness is really 'emotional illness' in other words, emotional pain or turmoil. Sometimes, simply being human means that we will experience emotional pain, some to a greater intensity than others. This does not necessarily mean that we are 'sick', or 'mentally ill'. The label 'mentally ill' needs a paradigm shift in description and perception. People who develop 'mental illness' (as it is currently described) are really hurting and emotionally fragile, as a result of real feelings and often abuse, neglect or damage of the heart of some kind. A miracle is a shift in perception, that is, when someone can see beyond their pain and start to change their thoughts. As the thoughts become more positive and helpful, then the cells and chemicals in the body automatically respond in a beneficial way, and behaviour and actions change for the better too. As part of this process, every little win only serves to promote further advancement, confidence and recovery. And, of course, if there is love and support from others during this process, it becomes so much easier.

It is not the 'emotionally ill' person's fault that they are unwell. The illness developed for a reason, and recovery is about trying to understand this, then doing something about it by trying to get well again to the best of one's ability. Often, the psychiatric medical model of treatment hinders this process because of the over-use and prolonged use of dangerous medications; when what the 'sick' person needs more is some rest, tender loving care, guidance, and opportunities for expressing feelings and emotions - to be validated, processed, and then come to terms with in a healthy way. Depending on how resilient a person may be, some people seem to be able to better handle more stress and hurt than others. However, the stronger among us have a duty as much as we can in our society today, to give a lot more help to the more vulnerable or less resilient who may have a mental illness. We are all unique, with different talents, interests and abilities; and it would not be right to consider any human being as 'lesser' or inferior. In this sense, we are really all equal, even though we are each individual and unique.

Our thoughts do actually create our reality. Quantum physics is starting to prove this. One needs to work from the inside (not outside), or from *within* to create their reality. The outside does not really influence us as much as we may think. We actually influence the outside. What happens to us, we actually attract- by the way we *think*. For example, if you think that you will not find that car park when you go to the shopping centre, you more than likely won't. However, if you believe and know that you will find that car parking space when you go to the shopping centre; you more than likely will. This is similar to the law of attraction and manifesting what happens to you by what you think about most. We can choose our thoughts, and once we realize that, miracles can happen (Foundation for Inner Peace, 1992).

Destructive emotions, such as hate, anger and fear, can erode our confidence and sense of happiness and well-being; and can act like poisons to the cells of the body and brain. This, in turn, can contribute to mental health problems or mental illness. The Dalai Lama remarked that:

Even though the vast majority of people experience negative emotions at various times, that does not mean that such emotions are inherent in the nature of mind. To give an example, when a hundred pieces of gold lie in a dusty place, all of them might be covered with dust, but that does not change the nature of gold itself. The belief, based on contemplative experiences, is that destructive emotions are not embedded in the basic nature of consciousness. Rather, they arise depending on circumstances and various habits and tendencies that express themselves from the outer core of consciousness (Goleman, *A Buddhist Psychology*, p.81, 2003).

To also assist in recovery, practicing *'mindfulness'*; living in the 'now' moment; can be very beneficial in helping someone who may have extremely bothersome thoughts, or may be under excessive stress, to 'go with the flow' more and just let go of other worries that really do not matter for the time being. It is important to keep your mind in the present and live in the present moment, doing one thing at a time. For example, if you are worrying, just worry; if you are reading, just read. Mindfulness is about *'not missing your own life'*; that is, what you do, and how you do it. You can only do one thing at a time if you are being mindful. It is the quality of attention and awareness of observing that matters in being mindful (Marsha Lineham PhD.).

Meditation and relaxation are also very good practices here for a lot of people, to help them to stay grounded and relieve stress. Therefore, this also can help one to train themselves out of unhealthy ways of thinking, and assist in maintaining healthy cell function and correcting any lack of necessary 'feel good' chemicals in the brain, when levels of neurotransmitters in the brain become depleted as a result of excessive stress or upset.

According to Deveson, where she explored the notion of *resilience*, with particular reference to families dealing with mental illness, she stated:

For quite a while, researchers tended to look at the big things that went wrong in people's lives - major traumas like war and death - but it is a culmination of adversities that does most harm - poverty, overcrowded homes, overcrowded schools, alcoholism or drug abuse, unemployment, sickness, separated families - a piling up of disasters which can damage the natural resilience of a child.

Many of the early theories about resilience focused on the role of genetics. Today, we know that although genes and personality are important, they are influenced by environment from the moment of conception. Who we are, and what happens to us, helps determine how we deal with life - whether we are vulnerable to anxiety and stress; whether we are inhibited or uninhibited; how we tackle adversities; how we interact with others. This notion of a dynamic interweaving of personality and environment is exciting because it means suddenly there are many points of possible intervention - from early childhood through to old age, all drawing upon the healing powers and adaptive resilience of the individual, strengthened by those environmental factors which might make a difference.

Hope is important; learning how to ask for help; humour; viewing ourselves and others in terms of strengths not weaknesses; and having some kind of meaning in life - which does not necessarily mean having a formal religion. Celebrated French writer, Colette, who was crippled by arthritis in old age, found meaning in the beauty that she saw in the very room in which she was confined. For those whose spirits are darkened through trauma or illness, this isn't always easy. But I have seen it happen, through friendship, through helping people feel needed, through listening, through acceptance, and through finding those things that bring joy in life.

The Seen But Forgotten

Ultimately, a sense of connectedness lies at the heart of resilience (Campbell et al, (eds), p. 24, Winter 2008)

Freud's account of the sexual nature of neuroses led him to develop a clinical treatment for treating such 'disorders'. This has become so influential, that when people think about psychoanalysis they often refer to this clinical treatment. The term: 'psychoanalysis' designates both the clinical treatment and the theory (as discussed in *PART II*) which underlies it. According to Thornton, the aim of the method may be stated simply in general terms, that is, to reestablish an harmonious relationship between the three elements which constitute the mind by uncovering and resolving unconscious repressed conflicts (Thornton, 2006).

The method of treatment pioneered by Freud grew out of Breuer's earlier discovery, where an 'hysterical' patient was encouraged to talk freely about the earliest instances of her symptoms and fantasies, the symptoms (supposedly) began to abate, and were totally eliminated when she was encouraged to remember the initial trauma which caused the symptoms. Moving away from his early attempts to explore the unconscious through hypnosis, Freud further developed this 'talking cure', acting on the assumption that the repressed conflicts were buried in the deepest recesses of the unconscious mind. Accordingly, Freud encouraged his patients to relax in a position in which they were deprived of strong sensory stimulation (hence, the couch scenario), even of keen awareness of the presence of the analyst. He then encouraged them to speak freely, preferably without much forethought, in the belief that he could then discern the unconscious forces which were hidden behind what was being said (Thornton, 2006).

If this style of therapy is conducive to recovery, and was successful in these earlier times, it begs the question then: why is it that today the practice of psychiatry involves, in many cases, the prescribing of dangerous drugs? Psychoanalysis, and especially Freud, have exerted a strong influence upon the popular imagination in the Western World over the past ninety years or so, and the theory and the practice of psychotherapy remain the object of a great deal of controversy. However, the practice of prescribing dangerous drugs is also the subject of controversy to many, and rightly so. The administering of dangerous and premature-death inducing chemicals as the major from of treatment for mental health issues and mental illness today is still a science in its infancy, with a long way to go in researching and producing much safer methods.

The debate which exists in relation to Freud is more rigorous than that relating to any other recent thinker (apart from, perhaps, Charles Darwin), with criticisms ranging from the supposition that Freud's theory was generated by logical confusions arising out of his alleged long-standing addiction to cocaine, to the view that he made an important, but grim, empirical discovery, which he knowingly suppressed in favor of the theory of the unconscious, because he thought that the latter would be more socially acceptable. His grim discovery was the widespread social prevalence of child sexual abuse, particularly in females (Thornton, 2006).

Eckhart Tolle wrote, in '*A New Earth: Awakening to Your Life's Purpose*':

The ego is in its essential nature pathological, if we use the word in its wider sense to denote dysfunction and suffering. Many mental disorders consist of the same egoic traits that operate in a normal person, except that they have become so pronounced that there pathological nature is now obvious to anyone, except the sufferer.

The mental illness that is called paranoid schizophrenia, or paranoid for short, is essentially an exaggerated form of ego. It usually consists of a fictitious story the mind has invented to make sense of a persistent underlying feeling of fear. The main element of the story is the belief that certain people (sometimes large numbers or almost everyone) are plotting against me, or are conspiring to control or kill me. The story often has an inner consistency and logic so that it sometimes fools others into believing it too. Sometimes organizations or entire nations have paranoid belief systems at their very basis. The ego's fear and distrust of other people, the tendency to emphasize the 'otherness' of others by focusing on their perceived faults and make those faults into their identity, is taken a little further and makes others into inhuman monsters. The ego needs others, but its dilemma is that deep down it hates and fears them. Jean-Paul Sartre's statement 'Hell is other people' is the voice of the ego. The person suffering from paranoia experiences that hell most acutely, but everyone in whom the egoic patterns still operate will feel it to some degree. The stronger the ego in you, the more likely it is that in your perception other people are the main source of problems in your life. It is also more than likely that you will make life difficult for others. But, of course, you won't be able to see that. It is always others who seem to be doing it to you (Tolle, 2005).

This view rings so true. Thus, for us to reducing the suffering which the ego can cause us, it is necessary to try to replace fear with *love*. The opposite of fear (or ego) is Love. The basic tenant, throughout history, of all religions (but which is not adhered to) is *love one another; or love your neighbour as you would also liked to be loved.* One cannot really base their life on religion, as such; as the amount of hypocrisy that has resulted out of most religions, has in itself created fear; as well as ending up being really about power and control. We just have to remember the Spanish Inquisition during the fourteenth century, where many innocent people, all over the Spanish-occupied world at that time, were tortured and murdered for being 'witches' or of the 'Devil' at the hands of the Catholic Church. The complete mindset of fear and paranoia at this time is a shocking example of what cruelty human beings are capable of when they set themselves up as being 'right' or 'holy'. In reality, the so-called 'men of the cloth' during the Inquisition who perpetrated this horror, were afraid and extremely egotistical. Hitler was also ego-driven and pathologically fearful. The Holocaust is another example of pseudo-religion, (pseudo-science as well in regards to Nazi psychiatrists during the Second World War), which led to terrible atrocities being inflicted upon innocent people. Still today, these types of occurrences happen in many parts of the world, but there is now an ever-greater awareness where people have 'had enough' and really want things to change for the better. There is a similar correlation here to the history of and the current practice of psychiatry, where it was and still is also about power and control, and atrocities inflicted upon vulnerable people in our society are committed.

It seems that we are all afraid to a certain degree. It will not be until we decide to truly co-operate and learn to love *ourselves*, that we are able to really love and appreciate *others*. We all go through pain at some time. There is no use in laying blame. If we blame our parents, it is important to realize that they did the best that they could, given the knowledge that they had at the time. It is not healthy to judge so much. Insanity can come from hatred, even hatred of one's parents or parent. The important thing is to learn from our experiences, and try to not make the same mistakes, so as not to repeat the cycle, and create a better future for ourselves (and others). The language spoken by Jesus still survives, and that of all the other great Masters as well - namely the likes of Buddha, Krishna, Mohammad, Yogananda, and Sai Baba and the Dalai Lama today. It is important for all of us to try to create a better world; then the instances of mental illness will become much less. This healing journey has to come from within, not without, in each one of us, as (as previously noted) we create our own reality - by our *thoughts*. No psychiatrist or drug can heal you. Healing has to come from within. Medications simply mask the emotional problems and distress and are simply a 'band aid' approach, even though they may initially be a necessary evil to help in times of intense suffering (where you hope like hell that they do not cause any adverse reactions and complicate things even further). However, to see the use of medications as a long-term solution is dangerous. By searching for meaning and purpose in life, for example, the soul can be re-awakened around mid-life, and one can truly then discover their life purpose, and help to create a new Earth. This can be a planet where peace exists and the presence of mental health problems and illnesses can be eliminated.

PART IX

CONCLUSION

As mentioned in *'PART II: Some Possible Causes of Mental Illness'*, according to Analytic Psychology and some other psychosocial theories, man seeks creative development, wholeness and completion. If this is suppressed by family and/or society in certain individuals, they can become so frustrated and upset that 'mental' (emotional) instability or illness could result. Upbringing, in some cases, society and its conflicting values and expectations, can lead to unfulfilment and despair in vulnerable individuals. Where some young people are suppressed and prevented from acting, within reason, according to their normal drives, this contributes to states of being upset, and excessive stressors which a young adult can experience when 'growing up' could tip an acutely sensitive or predisposed person into a mental (or nervous) breakdown. This is certainly something to be considered and admitted to by society and families, rather than immediately labeling someone as 'sick', when they could be having a normal response to an intolerable life situation.

If those individuals who have experienced mental illness and not recovered and still suffer psychological distress, can attempt to learn from their past, and even understand, perhaps, those who have hurt them; they could try to let go and *move on* from traumatic experiences of the past. Then, maybe they would be able to try to get better in touch with *who they really are* in their journey of recovery and growth.

One aspect of the psychiatric profession which still seems to exist in today's medical model of treatment of mental illness in the public hospital system (not so much in the private hospital system though) is an authoritarian form of psychotherapy, coupled with the use of dangerous drugs, where good counseling and therapy techniques are not employed, nor a person's real needs and problems listened to and taken into account. In addition, the use of modern 'anti-psychotic' drugs is still not the safest form of treatment, and they are often over-prescribed and used for too long periods of time for many people.

Admittedly, today's scientific knowledge in the field of psychiatry has progressed, especially since the late 1940's. However, chemical drug treatments still do not really work for a large proportion of people who suffer from mental illness, and relapses and rehospitalizations are numerous and common. In addition, funding for and research by the mainstream psychiatric associations and international drug companies is not headed in the right direction. One could also go so far as to say that compassion itself is often lacking. This is especially so in the public sector hospitals. And, anti-psychotic drugs are often forced upon people in the public mental health system, in Queensland (Australia), under the Queensland Mental health Act 2000, despite any adverse outcomes of concern. This should be made an illegal practice. It is actually a ludicrous and corrupt practice, and should not be allowed to happen by the medical profession in the public sector; by governments legislating against it. Social justice, basic human rights and personal freedom have been denied to many people with mental illness, not to mention the murders, suicides and other diseases inflicted on them because of modern psychiatric and pharmaceutical treatments. Some people with mental illness know that their medication is slowly killing them, and often refuse to take it. In some cases, they are forced by injection under a Mental Health Act, instead of the medical profession listening more to the reasons why a person is refusing medication and taking this into account in their 'treatment'.

Compassion is lacking from the society at large, basically because of a lack of understanding of and a lack of education about what it is like to have, or have had, a mental illness. For a person with a mental illness, being able to function at some level can only serve to increase their self-worth. Often, people with a psychotic disorder, for example, describe their lives as lonely, isolated and devoid of meaningful activity. With improved self-esteem and some nurturing and development of self love, and a better understanding from society as a whole, can come a lessening of such feelings as depression, anxiety, lack of motivation, and even tendencies towards paranoia.

For those who are lucky enough to experience a quicker recovery from a mental illness, perhaps years or even only months after, it is possible for the person to enter into a process of complete recovery and full wellness. In some instances, it has been possible for some people who have experienced a mental illness to be able to wean off their medication, or be maintained on a minimal dose and lead a more productive, happy and successful life after taking part in 'talk therapy' with a psychologist or counselor.

A more compassionate, more understanding and better-informed approach from society, the general public and some of the medical profession, towards those who suffer with mental illness is necessary in order for them to be able to have a better quality of life. Mental illness affects over twenty per cent of the population worldwide. Therefore, the stigma, fear and ignorance surrounding it: needs to be addressed by us; and everyone (including some mental health nurses, doctors and case managers); needs to better understand it. This is especially so in regards to the degree in which many people with mental illness really do suffer a lot of the time. This way, sufferers of mental illness can have a better quality of life, and have access to better treatments, and even have a chance at moving on and recovery. This would revolutionize the field of psychiatry and help change the direction of research and some of the views held by many psychiatrists (and the major drug companies), with regards to them admitting to the failures of modern drug treatments.

Psychiatrists would no longer need to be 'hood-winked' by the large drug companies, when they really start to care and be more open-minded to the truth, and cease being too scientific in their judgments. Of course, there does need to be objective evidence-based research in controlled trials and testing of drugs. However, where actually is the proof that they do know exactly which chemicals they are targeting, in the areas of the brain suspected to have an imbalance in the receptors.

Laurens van der Post, in "Jung and the Story of Our Time" (1976) wrote:

Compassion leaves an indelible blueprint of the recognition that life so sorely needs between one individual and another; one nation and another; one culture and another. It is also valid for the road which our spirit should be building now for crossing the historical abyss that still separates us from a truly contemporary vision of life, and the increase of life and meaning that awaits us in the future (Griffith, 1991).

The Seen But Forgotten

A more loving and compassionate approach in treating those suffering from mental illness is needed. Taking into account one's spiritual or religious beliefs would also go a long way towards better understanding and give more insight into an individual's state of mind or state of upset. By respecting these needs and treating the suffering person as an individual, with different views and beliefs, the mental health profession would advance and find even better approaches to help heal a person's body, mind and soul.

As suggested previously, some of the relief from the suffering and awful states of mind which can arise in psychosis or depressive illness, apart from medication at present, also needs to come from *within*. That is, by taking small steps in making efforts to help one self and by trying to work through extremely troubling thoughts and emotions with a good therapist. This is a very difficult task, and sadly, not everyone can do this successfully, for many reasons; particularly when there is no support or not enough help available.

Interestingly, some people who suffer with schizophrenia seem to have more than the average psychic and metaphysical interests, even abilities and talents, which they are both unaware and some aware of to a great degree. It seems even, at times, that they have access to different 'planes' which are not three dimensional with regards to the field of quantum physics. That is, they have access to another dimension; in other words, the 'fourth dimension'. They seem to have more interest than the average person in the 'afterlife' (or 'astral planes'): the other side of existence after this life on Earth, and can be occupied a lot with religious thinking. Perhaps this is because they are searching for meaning, during times of persistent fear, doubt and confusion? Of course, not all people with schizophrenia would have the same interests and ideas, as this depends on one's spiritual, religious and/or metaphysical beliefs, background, culture, education, et cetera.

It is also interesting to note, that some people who have experienced a psychotic break or 'flight from reason', have described it later on as a spiritual experience, a catalyst for transformation, or as an escape from a monotonous, boring or materialistic daily existence. Those who have recovered and been able to come out of psychosis, often experience true personal growth and an understanding that some psychiatrists and the drug companies refuse to want to know about, because then this could wreck a whole money-making industry of psychiatry and pharmaceutical treatments for mental illness. This is not common knowledge, but is a fact which they attempt to hide from the Western World. In addition, there have been cases where the drug companies falsify their results in double blind placebo-controlled trials in order to sell their drugs, with full knowledge that they are dangerous and can kill people, out of greed for more money. However, of course, this is not so in all cases of these studies and the outcomes and results of most of the research to date.

According to Berther (2007), in his writings on the *Treatment of Persons Assumed to be Suffering from a Mental Illness;* he stated that this entailed:-

(a) **Forced drug addiction**
(b) **Ethnic cleansing and genocide**
(c) **Imprisonment without trial**
(d) **Deaths in custody**
(e) **Deaths in the community**
(f) **Responsibility of government**
(g) **APOLOGY**

(h) *COMPENSATION*
(i) *REHABILITATION FOR SURVIVORS*

Berther also stated:

As I watched the apology to Aboriginal people on National Television, I wondered how much pressure is required to initiate an apology to mental health patients? During the last Federal election all parties either dismissed or ignored my pleas for a National Mental Health Act.

The Federal Government has shown very little interest in the genocide of a minority group of Australians (except for Kornelia Rau). She was also misdiagnosed by the Princess Alexandra Hospital! Only the media have attempted to bring the issues of mental health to the attention of both the public and governments. During the past six months, I have observed, read and heard a concentrated campaign on issues which cause assumed mental illness. Channel Seven and the ABC last night, 4BH Radio in all news slots yesterday, and the Courier Mail almost every second day; all combine to accentuate the problems of society that politicians have ignored since Noah built the Ark.

I have little knowledge of interstate systems, but I do have extensive first hand experience of the treatment of those assumed to have a mental illness in Queensland. Since 1995, I have been misdiagnosed, imprisoned without trial, forcibly injected with dangerous drugs; and observed at close hand the suicides of friends who were turned into drug addicts by the system. The hallucinatory nature of modern psychiatric drugs and overmedication causes: mania, depression, suicide, apparent mental illness, and in some extreme cases, violence and murder.

Despite the recent airing of a program on the sleeping pill 'Stilnox', the authorities chose to put a warning label on the product! They didn't even suspend its future use on new patients! The statement by the company that manufactured the product was more important than the evidence!

Politicians were teary-eyed about the treatment of Indigenous Australians by government. How about the deaths in custody, suicides and absolute wrecking of lives and careers by psychiatrists? Only forty years ago in Wolston Park, less than fifty per cent of patients survived the first twelve months of "TREATMENT"! Fifty-five years ago, the government employed European surgeons to perform LOBOTOMIES on patients in mental health institutions! Forty years ago, surgeons were still performing FULL HYSTERECTOMIES on teenage girls "assumed to be suffering from mental illness"! Was this a form of 'ethnic cleansing' originated by Adolf Hitler?

Today, authorized doctors, authorized nurses, and authorized security officers are still 'legally killing' persons assumed to be suffering from a mental illness. Today 'Dual Diagnosis' allows criminals to evade judicial process, and hide in Authorized Mental Health Service Facilities. Today, flawed and inept legislation is an excuse for government employees to do literally anything to anybody, under cover of "assumed mental illness". Today, the legalities of current legislation mean nothing to psychiatrists, nurses, doctors, security officers and administrators. When is the Queensland Government going to prosecute those responsible for brutality and genocide? When is Australia going to have a NATIONAL MENTAL HEALTH ACT (in keeping with World Health Organization Guidelines)?

The Seen But Forgotten

When is the Federal Government going to issue an APOLOGY and provide appropriate COMPENSATION to the survivors of institutional treatment? (Kornelia Rau looks like getting some). When is Australia going to reject the international drug companies' products and outlandish claims? When are we going to admit that all drugs cause side-effects, and that individuals all have different physiology, with different reactions to drugs? You can't treat people like a herd of sheep. Don't assume that all are stupid! Queensland is euthanasing some of the most brilliant minds in our society! When is Queensland going to establish a major REHABILITATION FACILITY FOR VICTIMS? There is three thousand acres of government land available at 'The Park', (a fitting memorial to all those who died there)! (Berther, 2007).

According to Berther, the old attitudes still exist. Assume that every patient has a mental illness and experiment on them with drugs. Psychiatry has no proven basics in medicine. Drug theory is at best simply experimental, depending on whether you get a positive or negative reaction. Academics write theories and extensive reports on trials of drugs, which are usually large scale experiments controlled by vested interests (the drug producing companies); and which are performed on victims whose brains have, in many cases, already been 'fried' by other dangerous drugs.

Berther noted also:

Why not do your double-blind controlled trials on psychiatrists and normal people, and find out what percentage of 'trialees' can be "created" into people with "apparent mental illness"? Experimentation is needed to keep up the numbers of patients required to justify the theory of modern psychiatric practices which allows some "doctors" to "work" in a branch of "medicine" where there is no proven basics of fact, and no accountability. "THE CAUSE?" Get to the cause and fix it! All prospective psychiatric registrars need to be psychologically tested before getting "a license to experiment on patients". If the killer drugs don't work, don't use them! If your proposed treatment has no medical basis, don't use it! Train psychologists to treat the "cause of mental illness". Don't fry patients' brains with drugs to hide the problems of society. Don't protect criminals by classifying them as "psych patients". Only some instances may be applicable. Everybody, given the conditions of pressure and provocation, is capable of killing under extreme stress. But, drug addicts and alcoholics who choose to bow to peer pressure and fry their brains are not the true sufferers of mental illness. Treat the cause! Don't "experiment with the symptoms".

Don't make hospital security officers capture patients and hold them down for nurses to inject with killer drugs. They also are aware of the results of modern psychiatric treatment. Don't jam up psychiatric institutions with drug addicts and alcoholics and criminals hiding from due legal process. Free up beds to treat the schizophrenics and sexual abuse victims who are the "genuine" mental health consumers. They need the most help. They shouldn't be turned away from assessment centres and "sent home" to suicide or attack others. This is the twenty-first century! Overhaul "the System". Reinstate the checks and balances of MHA 1974 without Section 69. Restore liability to keep the experimenters honest when using "laboratory rats". Don't "create mental illness" just to keep "doctors" in work.

Encourage psychologists to treat the cause, with as few drugs as possible. They must be astute enough to distinguish between the "manipulating child" and the "actual victim of mental and sexual abuse" (Berther, 2007).

It was stated earlier in *PART II*, that the ego's job was to satisfy the id's impulses, not offend the morals of the super-ego, while still taking into consideration the reality of a situation. This, obviously, for all of us is not an easy thing to accomplish. We do not want either the id or the super-ego to be too dominant, so we speak to both of them, try to listen to each perspective, and then make a decision. According to analytic psychology, this decision is the ego talking, that is, that part of the mind looking for that healthy balance. With an illness like schizophrenia, this job is difficult, as the mind is 'split', and perhaps some of the ego defence mechanisms are faulty. The ego has a difficult time satisfying both the id and the super-ego, even though it does not have to do this without help. Ego defenses, such as repression, regression and projection, are tools which it can use to help in its job as a mediator and which help defend the ego when it has a difficult time making both the id and the super-ego happy. When these defence mechanisms become too strong, for example with excessive tendencies for projection, this can lead to unhealthy thoughts and behaviour, such as paranoia. One could also comment that the ego has become weak due to environmental triggers, such as where an individual was subject to suppression or some kind of prolonged abuse as a child.

The existence of schizophrenia may not be as biological or physical in origin as currently thought. The psychological world; spiritual beliefs; experiences; background; even illicit drug use; in combination with genes, are all contributing factors. The chemical imbalance may occur as a result of environment, trauma and background, more so than currently believed. And, as the label of 'schizophrenia' covers a spectrum of disorders of the illness, the different possible triggering factors mentioned in *PART II* could account for such differences in the experiences of the illness in different individuals. It could be said, too, that the experience of hearing voices, in any mental illness, can occur when a person is in internal conflict and *at war with themselves*; and totally preoccupied with their own thoughts in the mind. Perhaps, here, they are actually attempting to get in touch with their *inner self* or real self, and separate out what is *not* them. For example, when there is conflict occurring, perhaps as a result of old limiting beliefs and values adopted from society or family which no longer suit them and *who they are*. They could be attempting to 'tear the world' out of their system in order to try to ask '*Who Am I?*' This could be as a result of emotional shocks, or conditioning in childhood, differing values to those of one's parents and family, leading to confusion, alienation at times, victimization, shame, inner turmoil, extreme anger, intense fighting and arguments, a tendency to lay blame too much, and all sorts of other upsetting events and dysfunction.

Auditory hallucinations come from a state of mind resulting from too much stress, or extreme fatigue, drugs, suppression, intense conflicts; and their content can be about one's worst *fears* coming to the fore in one's mind. The hearing of voices, especially so in schizophrenia, may only be able to dissipate or cease when the person tries to 'find him or herself', and eventually learn, find out or try to practice ways to grow and let go of anger, hurt, frustration and fear. This process can, and probably would, take many years and require a certain amount of maturity. These feelings and thoughts are actually a part of a *state of mind*. One can even try to forgive (not forget), but does not really have to forgive, as here a serious dilemma can arise. It is important for the person to be aware not to fool themselves. That is, if they cannot truly forgive, then do not pretend to do it, or recovery cannot take place.

Constant rumination over past hurts and traumas is not good for anyone's mental state, or physical health. Remembering and then learning from one's past is a much more positive way to try to help one self and others, and much more likely to promote recovery where there may be mental illness. Obviously, this is more easily said than done, and can take a long time. Also, learning to *love oneself* despite our faults can bring a happier and more confident state of being, which influences thoughts, emotions and behaviour in a positive way. And, ultimately taking control back of one's life, and in some cases, moving away from controlling or narcissistic people, can give one more time to heal and avoid any further abuse or 'guilt trips' put onto them, if this had been happening.

Young people who develop schizophrenia, for some reason, seem to have a greater tendency to being frail, very sensitive and more vulnerable than the average 'normal' person. It seems that in late teens or early adulthood, various normal stressors in life are enough to tip such a sensitive person into emotional and psychological breakdown more easily than others. They seem to have greater sensitivities and great imaginations, yet they are often misunderstood.

Sensitive people who are susceptible to developing schizophrenia and the like of weakening of states of mind and dissociation from self, are the types of people who may need to educate the three-dimensional 'normal' people about the value they can offer society. Rather than a person with schizophrenia accepting feelings of shame, that are often forced upon them from a young age, perhaps due to teasing, or cruelty imposed on them by their peers, parents, or other groups for being 'different', they can know that every time they criticized for being extra-ordinary, they can grow stronger against the ordinary person who cares not to seek meaning and purpose in life. The truth is, many 'normal' people are brought up to kill their senses by their parents or social circles, and taught to ignore their gifts and believe that their senses (or sensitivities) are not important (Jacqueline Musgrave, 2005).

Often, many 'normal' people fight, and are competitive with others in a really jealous way because they know not how to find their own genius. As a result, they try to 'stamp out' the sensitive or artistic 'schizophrenic' person, with little regard for the consequences or the true well being of such a person. Once a schizophrenic person gives themselves the right to validate themselves, they can cease to be affected by the jealous populous, who think that they are 'normal' and have all of the answers, simply because three-dimensional objectivity and 'logic' says that it is so (Jacqueline Musgrave, 2005).

Without the sensitive people, the world would lack soul, compassion and art. This is why it is so important for the sensitive individuals to believe in themselves and their, sometimes extra-ordinary, abilities, so that they can attempt to also become leaders in our world, which is currently dominated by materialistic, wooden dummies. There is too much abuse, famine and war to justify our current leaders and societal rules and structures, as well as many individuals' self-centeredness and greed. Some sensitive souls could be helped to realize their 'specialness', so that they may be engaged in helping to bring about change in the world, and help to make it a more peaceful and meaningful place in which to live.

All illness stems from a *state of mind*. This includes both physical illness and mental illness. The great Chinese sages and Indian philosophers knew this, thousands of years ago. Processing hurts and moving forward by trying to *let go* of 'baggage' and not 'live in the past', and coming to terms with and gaining an understanding of one's history (to date) and life path, can be very healing itself for damaged people, or people who are stuck. Then trying to turn things around, even start over, and make the best of a tough situation by *moving on* and creating the best new life you can for yourself, is a very good way of becoming 'successful', even then helping others who also may be in a similar situation to that which you once were. One can ask *'What is success for me?'* It may not be only once you have that new car or new house; or identifying with an outside measure of social standing. It will more than likely be when you are *happy*, and then all the rest will automatically come. You will have a right, too, to experience peace, harmony, love, beauty, prosperity and abundance; as we all do. Doors will open the more you engage with others, and opportunities will come knocking.

It is possible to *fight your way* out of a mental illness, by continually learning, studying and working towards your goals; and by not becoming a passive victim of modern psychiatry. It is such a tragic outcome where so many people have either thrown away, or had their life stolen away from them, because of the rigid, tunnel vision-style thinking of the field of psychiatry in the public health sector and the large pharmaceutical industry towards people who develop mental illness. This has really got to change. It has to stop. Too many people are dying before their time, or suiciding, because of the current medical treatments for mental illness; and the lack of resources available to truly help those who are experiencing symptoms of mental illness, and who tragically 'fall through the cracks' of a mental health system which is unable to meet demand.

Some things are improbable, but, all things are possible

APPENDIX

SPIRITUALITY – THE MISSING LINK IN PSYCHIATRY

(Adapted from Griffith, 1991)

SUMMARY

WHY NOT COMBINE THE TWO IN SEARCHING FOR ANSWERS?
OUR HISTORY HAS SHOWN THAT EXTREMES HAVE ALWAYS CREATED PROBLEMS

PSYCHIATRY IS A SCHOOL OF THOUGHT LACKING IN BALANCE, AS IT DENIES MANY SPIRITUAL QUESTIONS AND THEIR MEANING FOR LIFE ITSELF BY BEING TOO MECHANISTIC

HEART	HEAD
HOLISTIC SUBJECTIVE INTROSPECTION Vs.	**MECHANISTIC OBJECTIVE SCIENCE**
Our psyche or soul or life force i.e. those activities of the self in search of guidance, wholeness and completion, projected onto the world experience	our ego i.e. those activities of the brain which express themselves in intelligent actions
(Jungian)	(Freudian)

127

SPIRITUALITY	Vs.	PSYCHIATRY
Conscious thought searching for meaning, relying on subjective feelings and experience, as well as subconscious factors such as Intuition		Conscious thought searching for knowledge, proof and cause of our upset

The word 'psychiatry' comes from the Greek 'psyche': which means 'soul', and 'iatreia': This means 'healing'- literally meaning 'soul healing'. Perhaps the medical model of today's practice of psychiatry should look more deeply into the importance of people's spiritual beliefs, experiences and problems?

Jeremy Griffith wrote, in *'Beyond the Human Condition'*:

In order to disarm our states of upset it has been necessary to explain what we have only been able to feel. The expression of frustrated and, at times, exalted (momentarily relieved) ego associated with the human condition are clear from looking at our history. Our soul, in all its forms, has not been attacked and repressed without reason.

While seeking knowledge, science had to evade integrative ideals because they unjustly criticized our divisive upset state. We had to be free from the integrative ideals to search for understanding of those ideals. This also meant that science had to avoid subjective introspection and depend only on objective research. We had to be free from the condemning integrative ideals that our conscience insisted on.

If the truth *is revealed, the next task would be to have everyone confront it. Humanity's 'brave new world' is the journey into self to liberate our repressed psyche or soul* (Griffith, 1991).

Victoria Musgrave

Wisdom from the Dalai Lama

Meditations on the Family

The levels of understanding and respect found in traditional societies are often dictated by the survival conditions, and contentment also depends on temporary ignorance of other possible ways of life. Ask Tibetan nomads if they would prefer to be better protected from the winter cold, if they would like stoves that did not blacken the inside of the tents, if they would like to be better cared for when they are ill, or if they would be interested to see what is happening on the other side of the world by means of television. I know exactly what they would answer.

Economic and technological progress is desirable and necessary. It is the culmination of many factors so complex that they escape us and it would be naïve to think that we can solve all our problems simply by halting progress. However, it definitely should not take place haphazardly. It should go hand in hand with the development of moral values. It is our responsibility as human beings to ensure that these two tasks are accomplished simultaneously. This is the key to our future. A society in which material development co-exists with spiritual progress is one where true happiness is really possible.

REFERENCES

Alcohol and Drug Information Service (Handout), **About Withdrawal and its Symptoms-What is Happening to Me?** Brisbane, Australia, 2003.

AllPsych and Heffner Media Group, Inc., **Ego Defense Mechanisms in Psychology 101**, www.allpsych.com/psychology101/defenses.html, 2004.

Beattie, M., **The Language of Letting Go**, Hazelden Information and Educational Services, Hazelden Foundation, United States of America, 1990.

Bullock, A., Stallybrass, O. (eds), **The Fontana Dictionary of Modern Thought,** Fontana Books, London, 1997.

Campbell, H., Spencer, D. (eds), **Remembering Goodna,** 'Balance', the Journal of the Mental Health Association (Qld) Inc., Australia, Summer 2008, pp24-25.

Campbell, H., Spencer, D. (eds), **The Importance of Resilience in Helping People Deal With Adversity**, 'Balance', the Journal of the Mental Health Association (Qld) Inc., Australia, Winter 2008, p.24.

Canadian Mental Health Association Website, **Meaning of Mental Health,** www.cmha.ca, 2008.

Dornan, D., **Mental Health Recovery: What Helps and What Hinders?**, National Alliance for the Mentally Ill Website, Santa Cruz County, (NAMI SCC), www.namiscc.org, 2005.

Foundation for Inner Peace, **A Course in Miracles**, Foundation for Inner peace, Mill Valley CA, 1992.

Goleman, D., The Dalai Lama, **Destructive Emotions and How We Can Overcome Them,** Bloomsbury, Great Britain, 2003.

Goleman, D., **Emotional Intelligence – Why it Can Matter More Than IQ,** Bloomsbury, London, 1996.

Griffith, J., **Beyond the Human Condition**, Foundation for Humanity's Adulthood, Sydney, Australia, 1991.

Hillard, E. B., **Manic Depressive Illness – An Information Book for Patients, Their Families and Friends,** Royal Columbian Hospital, New West Minister, B.C Winter, Internet, 1992.

Hillman, J., **The Souls Code: In Search of Character and Calling**, Random House Inc., New York, Australia, 1996.

Huskey, A., **Partners in Recovery Adult System of Care Conference 2000,** National Alliance for the Mentally Ill, Santa Cruz County (NAMI SCC), www.namiscc.org/newsletters, 2005.

Lewinsohn, P.M., Munoz, R.F., Youngren, M.A., Ziess, A.M., **Control Your Depression,** Prentice Hall Press, New York, 1986.

London Health Observatory Website, **Disease Groups-Mental Health Overview and Definitions**, www.lho.org.uk, 2008.

Mental Health Western Australia, Department of Health, **What is Mental Health?**, www.health.wa.gov.au, 2008.

National Mental Health Information Centre, online publication, **Before You Label People, Look at Their Contents,** www.mentalhealth.org, 2008.

Newsletter, the Schizophrenia Fellowship of Queensland Inc., **The Sunday Mail Highlights Mental Health Advances: Headlines, Schizophrenia Research Institute,** August 2007, p1, p7.

Rose, S. P. (ed), Princeton, N.J., **From Brains to Consciousness? Essays on the New Sciences of the Mind,** Allen Lane, The Penguin Press, Princeton University Press, 1998.

Schizophrenia.com, NARSAD, The Mental Health Association, **Schizophrenia Daily News Blog,** www.narsad.org, October 05, 2007.

Stevens, J., **Neo-alchemy and the Meaningful Life**, Sumeria Press, first published 1994.

Taylor, A., Sluckin, W., Davies, D.R., Reason, J.T., Thomson, R., Colman, A.M., **Introducing Psychology,** 2nd Edition, Penguin Books, Harmondsworth, 1982.

The Main Place: Your Place to Recover, Mental Health Recovery Center, Internet, Ohio, www.themainplace.org/. 2008.

Thornton, S.P., **Sigmund Freud,** Internet Encyclopedia of Philosophy, www.iep.utm.edu, 2006.

Tolle, E., **A New Earth: Awakening to Your Life's Purpose**, Michael Joseph Limited, Penguin Books, Victoria, Australia, Canada, New York, USA, London,

England, New Delhi, India, Auckland, New Zealand, Johannesburg, South Africa, 2005.

Wilkie, W., **Understanding Stress Breakdown**, Greenhouse Publications, Richmond, Victoria, Australia, 1985.

www.ingramcontent.com/pod-product-compliance
Lightning Source LLC
Chambersburg PA
CBHW031211270326
41931CB00006B/516